Insuring Children's Health

Insuring Children's Health

Contentious Politics and Public Policy

Alice Sardell

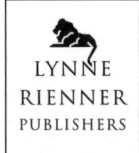

LYNNE
RIENNER
PUBLISHERS

BOULDER
LONDON

Published in the United States of America in 2014 by
Lynne Rienner Publishers, Inc.
1800 30th Street, Boulder, Colorado 80301
www.rienner.com

and in the United Kingdom by
Lynne Rienner Publishers, Inc.
3 Henrietta Street, Covent Garden, London WC2E 8LU

© 2014 by Lynne Rienner Publishers, Inc. All rights reserved

Library of Congress Cataloging-in-Publication Data
Sardell, Alice, author.
  Insuring children's health : contentious politics and public policy /
Alice Sardell.
       pages cm
  Includes bibliographical references and index.
  ISBN 978-1-62637-035-7 (hc : alk. paper)
  1. Child health services—Government policy—United States. 2. Child health insurance—United States. 3. Poor children—Medical care—Government policy—United States. 4. Health services accessibility—United States.
I. Title.
  RJ102.S27 2014
  368.38'20083—dc23

                                                              2013042269

British Cataloguing in Publication Data
A Cataloguing in Publication record for this book
is available from the British Library.

Printed and bound in the United States of America

The paper used in this publication meets the requirements
of the American National Standard for Permanence of
Paper for Printed Library Materials Z39.48-1992.

5   4   3   2   1

*To the policy entrepreneurs
who made an expansion of health insurance
for US children possible
through their commitment and skill*

*To Martin Eisenberg (1940–2013),
who lived his commitment to social justice every day*

Contents

Acknowledgments		ix
1	Policy Frameworks and Children's Health	1
2	The Emergence of the Child Health Advocacy Community	25
3	Policy Legacies and Political Entrepreneurs: Enacting Children's Health Insurance	49
4	Ideological Conflict over a "Bipartisan" Program	79
5	Expanding the Program: Advocacy and Framing	105
6	The State of Children's Health	137
List of Acronyms		155
References		157
Index		171
About the Book		183

Acknowledgments

I am indebted to all of the people I interviewed during the course of my research. All were extremely generous with information and insights during their very busy workdays. Their descriptions of meetings, hearings, conversations, legislative actions, and relationships and their thoughts about them were central to my understanding of the policy processes detailed in this book.

I would like to express my gratitude to the Professional Staff Congress–City University of New York Research Award Program, which supported my research on child health policy with five grant awards between 1995 and 2009; to Queens College for a Presidential Research Award, which provided a full semester of research time; and to Donald Scott, former dean of social sciences, and Leonard Rodberg, chair of the Department of Urban Studies, at Queens College for their long-term support of my work.

I was a recipient of the Robert Wood Johnson Foundation Investigator Award in Health Policy Research Program from 1999 to 2003. In addition to the very generous financial support it provided, the program sponsored conferences and meetings at which awardees presented their research and worked together on joint projects. The level of intellectual discourse about health policy and US politics and society, as well as the spirit of camaraderie at these meetings, was unmatched in my professional life. I wish to thank the staff of the Investigator Awards Program as well as my fellow awardees for that wonderful experience.

Alison Kanosky did wonderful work in assisting with my analysis of frames used in congressional hearings; I know that she will be publishing her own research on US sociocultural history very soon.

I was very lucky to have my manuscript carefully read by two anonymous reviewers whose comments were both extremely kind and extremely useful. William Gormley shared his wise thoughts on the framing section of Chapter 5.

I would like to thank David Nexon for the generous access that he granted me to the State Children's Health Insurance Program files in the office of Senator Edward Kennedy in 1998, Craig Ramsay for giving me his research material on the National Association of Children's Hospitals and Related Institutions and the March of Dimes, and Sara Rosenbaum for sharing her 1988 manuscript on Medicaid expansion. Librarians Dorothy M. Attridge and Astrid Emel of the Rittenberg Law Library of St. John's University School of Law were very hospitable during the weeks that I used their library as a guest.

Many thanks are due to Lawrence D. Brown, who first suggested to me that I research the issue of children's health policy for a special issue of the *Journal of Health Politics, Policy, and Law* in 1990 and who was very appreciative of the product; and to Sally Cohen, Bonnie Lefkowitz, Jane Levitt, James Morone, Thomas Oliver, and Frank Thompson, who have been supportive and sharing colleagues in health policy and politics over the years.

My thanks go to friends and colleagues who were interested and encouraging during the years of work on all phases of this project: Peter Beitchman, Laura Davis, Cristina DiMeo, Martin Eisenberg, Ginny Fox, Tarry Hum, Claire Jacobsohn, Mahulika Khandalwal, William Muraskin, and Stephen Steinberg. And to my friend Nicholas Irons, who could always be counted on to teach me what I needed to know about my computer.

I am very grateful to Alyssa Gillego, Joseph Dayan, and Andrew Evans of Beth Israel Medical Center, who showed me that the very latest medical knowledge and the highest level of clinical skill can beautifully coexist with a caring and nurturing relationship with their patients, one in which patients are fully equal partners in the health-care decisionmaking process.

One of the most pleasurable aspects of preparing the final version of this book was talking with Jessica Gribble, superb acquisitions editor at Lynne Rienner Publishers. Jessica knows a great deal about writing, about publishing books on politics and policy, and about a lot more.

I want to thank my daughters, Molly and Rachel Catchen, who have given me enormous joy and an intense interest in how US children's lives could be made better.

In spite of all of the support that enabled me to research and write this book, the final responsibility for its contents is mine.

1

Policy Frameworks and Children's Health

The policy processes that led to the expansion of US children's health insurance were imbued with tragedy, drama, and irony. Tragedy occurred with the death of Deamonte Driver, a twelve-year-old Maryland boy who died on February 25, 2007, after surgery for a brain infection that originated in an abscessed tooth that had not been treated. This tragedy brought media attention and a swift response from members of Congress—first a hearing and then legislation expanding publicly funded dental-care coverage for children. But behind this story is another very important story that helped make the congressional response to the tragedy of Deamonte's death possible.

That is the story of the Children's Dental Health Project, an advocacy group created a decade earlier by a "policy entrepreneur" concerned about the enormity of the problem of lack of access to dental care for low-income children. A dramatic, sometimes tragic event occurs and the media and elected officials respond; this response is a very common phenomenon in US public policymaking. But these dramas are not the most important part of the process of creating policy. Instead it is the policy research, the dissemination and discussion of that research, and the development of relationships between outside advocates and elected and appointed officials over time that establish the ideas that become policy responses to dramatic events. Through this book, I tell the story of the individuals and groups that were critical to increasing health insurance coverage for US children from the 1980s through 2009.

I begin that story with two other politically dramatic events—presidential vetoes that highlight the ideological conflict that attended the discussion of the expansion of federal health insurance coverage for children when the State Children's Health Insurance Program (SCHIP), created in 1997, was due to be reauthorized. On October 3, 2007, and then again on December 12, President George W. Bush vetoed an expansion and reauthorization of SCHIP that had been passed by large majorities in Congress. Bush opposed the legislation even though many business groups, including insurance and pharmaceutical companies, supported it, as did key Republican health leaders in the Senate and, according to polls, more than two-thirds of the US population.

When SCHIP was created, conservative Republicans controlled Congress. Republican support reflected the fact that SCHIP was not an "entitlement program," as is Medicaid, but rather a federal block grant to the states. So it is ironic that a Republican president twice vetoed a children's health insurance program that at its inception was hailed by Republican governors and Republican congressional leaders as a victory for state autonomy in health policy.

The United States has a much higher infant mortality rate and a lower rate of childhood immunization than other wealthy, postindustrial nations. Assuring that children in the United States have health insurance coverage would appear to be a noncontroversial, consensual, and even a popular issue, the latter confirmed by public opinion polls. Yet the policy history of children's health insurance is marked by drama and controversy. Both its supporters and opponents have viewed it in terms of the larger issue of universal coverage, and its fate has been linked to major electoral change. SCHIP was not reauthorized until Barack Obama became president. On February 4, 2009, during his third week in office, President Obama signed the same legislation, with minor changes, that Bush had vetoed.

In this book, I examine the political debates and dramas surrounding this issue. I explain how a child health "policy community" emerged in the 1980s and focused on the expansion of Medicaid eligibility for pregnant women and children, how children's health insurance moved to the top of the policy agenda in the late 1990s, then how a liberal Democratic senator and a conservative Republican senator partnered with the premier children's advocacy group to push a new children's health insurance initiative through a Republican Congress.

I also discuss how the policy process itself shaped the characteristics of SCHIP.

I then focus on the new set of issues raised when SCHIP came up for reauthorization ten years later: whether parents of eligible children, pregnant women, and legal immigrant children should be included in the program; the services that should be mandated by the federal government; the cost of the program; and how high income levels for eligibility should go. Legislative provisions that would expand SCHIP in several ways led President Bush and other conservative Republicans to oppose the program for ideological reasons. One Republican senator (Tom Coburn, OK) called it "part of an effort to bring everyone into a socialized health care system" (Pear 2007).

SCHIP is significant as a policy, and its policy history is a significant case for analysis. SCHIP was the first major piece of federal legislation to establish a separate health insurance program for children; it has helped to reduce inequality in access to health care. The Balanced Budget and Revenue Reconciliation Acts of 1997, which authorized the program, allocated the largest amount of federal money to children's health since the passage of Medicaid three decades earlier (Pear 1997c). As a consequence of the implementation of the SCHIP legislation, the proportion of low-income uninsured children had decreased by one-third between 1997 and 2005 (Mann 2007) while the proportion of uninsured adults increased.

Good health is critical to the ability of children to develop and to learn. An argument made as early as the 1980s—that investment in children's health care will reduce future health costs—is increasingly salient as we face enormously high health-care costs and compelling health-care problems such as childhood obesity and rising rates of mental illness in children and adolescents. In addition, there is growing scientific evidence that many adult health conditions originate in childhood (Halfon, DuPlessis, and Inkelas 2007).

The 1997 enactment of SCHIP and its 2009 reauthorization illuminate important aspects of the broader debate about the US health-care system. SCHIP was created after the failure of the Clinton administration's health reform plan. For congressional Democrats and some advocates for universal coverage, it was viewed as an incremental step in achieving broader coverage. For state governors, particularly Republican governors, the structure of SCHIP was a victory for the states within the federal and state health policy relationship.

Typically, a program's reauthorization is a routine matter because it is viewed as "distributive": having benefits for some groups, but few costs for others.[1] This was not the case with SCHIP reauthorization. There was wide bipartisan support for the program during the years of its implementation and when it was due to be reauthorized in 2007; a broad coalition of both health industry groups and consumer advocates was supportive. Yet the program's reauthorization was filled with partisan and ideological conflict.

The effort to expand SCHIP had stimulated a historical ideological controversy about the relative roles of the public and the private sectors in the US health-care system that has reoccurred several times since the late nineteenth century (see Sardell 1988: ch. 2). Thus, to supporters of expanding public health insurance coverage, SCHIP expansion was a positive first step; to opponents of expanding coverage, SCHIP was a "Trojan horse" that would bring forth a system of universal public health insurance. This long-standing ideological debate over the US health-care system occurred within the context of the increased ideological polarization between the Democratic and Republican parties.

Children and childhood have special meaning within the context of US social policy. Babies and children, especially young children, are viewed as both vulnerable and innocent. They are "constructed" as unformed and malleable; they are not yet what they will become. They are thus more "fixable" than adults (Sardell 1991) and have a "dual status" as existing in both the present and the future (Mayall 1998). Children are therefore outside of the paradigm of the moral distinction between the "worthy" and the "unworthy" and the powerful notions of "us" and "them" that have historically been central to US social policy (Katz 1983; Morone 2003). Yet the case of children's health insurance also reinforces the central importance of framing strategies in successful policy enactment, particularly when the target populations are those without political resources of their own. Children's innocence and our moral obligation to the vulnerable was not enough; children's health insurance was framed as a "cost-effective" program for the children of "hard-working parents."

In addition to explaining SCHIP as a product of the politics of US children's policy and the politics of health insurance policy, I also provide lessons about the politics of US social policy more generally. An analysis of the policy processes related to the expansion of health insurance coverage for US children *over time* provides important insights into the dynamics of the policy process itself. Relationships between and among policy actors in and outside of government, advocacy strategies, and the linkages between a series of policy events are all clarified by using a longitudinal lens. A comparison of the creation of SCHIP in

1997 and the reauthorization process in 2007–2009 enables me to analyze changes in the child health policy community over time, the way in which the issue of children's health coverage was framed at the program's creation and then ten years later, and the intersection of policy activity by advocates with changes in the larger political environment.

Insuring Children's Health is the first book in which policy theories and frameworks are used to analyze the politics of children's health insurance over time. The analysis of federal policymaking on "children's issues" and the potential for mobilizing around such issues other than health care has received attention from political scientists (Skocpol 1992; Gormley 1995; Cohen 2001; Skocpol and Dickert 2001; Imig 1996, 2001, 2006; Crowley 2003). Since children themselves are not political actors and have no political resources, a key strategy in political advocacy for children is "framing." William T. Gormley Jr. (2012) examines the framing strategies of various policy actors at both the national and state levels across several policy domains, including child health. But to date, there have been only a few scholarly articles focusing exclusively on the national politics of children's health policy (Sardell 1991; Sardell and Johnson 1998; Brandon, Chaudry, and Sardell 2001; Rosenbaum and Sonosky 2001; Oberlander and Lyons 2009).

There is health policy literature that has examined the implementation of SCHIP in terms of programmatic issues such as enrollment barriers and the substitution of public for private insurance. (I will be referring to this literature in Chapters 4 and 6.) Scholars have also analyzed the contemporary child health system and made important proposals for improvement (see, for example, Grason and Guyer 1995; Stein 1997; Halfon, DuPlessis, and Inkelas 2007; Rosenbaum 2008). Although these are critical contributions to the policy discussion of how to improve the health of US children, they do not examine the policy processes through which these proposals are presented and considered, adopted, or rejected, nor do they examine the roles of various actors, their interactions, and the broader political and social environment in which these interactions occur.

In contrast, there are several major studies of the political processes that produced Medicare policy (Marmor 2000; Jacobs 1993; Himelfarb 1995; Oberlander 2003) that failed to produce national health insurance in the United States (Jacobs 1993; Skocpol 1997; Hacker 2002; Quadagno 2005), and that resulted in the creation of the Affordable Care Act (Starr 2011; McDonough 2011; Altman and Shactman 2011). The politics of the Medicaid program are intimately connected to children's health insurance, although children are only one of the constituency groups served by Medicaid. The majority of publicly insured children are enrolled in Medicaid, and the origins of SCHIP/CHIP are rooted in the federal politics of Medicaid. Stevens and Stevens (1974), Smith (2002), Grogan and Patashnik (2003), Olson (2010), and Thompson (2012) present comprehensive, important discussions of the policy history of Medicaid.[2] Frank Thompson applies his rich analysis of the challenges of program administration within the complex federal health care system to SCHIP as well as Medicaid.

In this first chapter, I discuss the theoretical frameworks used to illuminate the very fluid and complicated policy processes that led to the creation and expansion of a federal children's health insurance program in the United States and briefly outline the way that interviews were conducted with participants in these processes. I will then place these events within a larger historical and ideological context by outlining the politics of federal funding for maternal and child health programs from the early twentieth century through the 1970s.

Policy Frameworks

The policy frameworks that are most useful in understanding the dynamics of new program creation, as well as program expansion, in the US context are John Kingdon's policy streams model (1995) and Mark A. Peterson's discussion (1997) of how "policy legacies" shape current policy actions. The advocacy coalition framework developed by Paul Sabatier (1988) refines the critical but general concept of policy networks. Anne Schneider and Helen Ingram's work (1993) on the social construction of target populations and the related interdisciplinary literature on "framing" are also central to understanding the policy process for a population such as children.

Kingdon's Model of the Policy Process

Kingdon's policy streams model provides a comprehensive and dynamic theoretical framework for analyzing the US policy process. Included in his model are the way that issues are defined (or "framed"), the role of ideas and values in the policy process, and the activities and interrelationships of a wide variety of public and private actors. Kingdon's focus is the question of why particular issues get on the governmental agenda at specific points in time; but it is also helpful in conceptualizing the process of policy formulation (see Zahariadis 1996; Sardell and Johnson 1998). My analysis of the creation of the State Children's Health Insurance Program (presented in Chapter 3) draws on Kingdon's framework as well as others to be discussed later.

The strength and usefulness of this framework is its conceptualization of three different "streams" of policy-relevant activity that can go on simultaneously, in contrast to a linear model of a series of policy stages. The three streams are the "problem stream," the "policy stream," and the "politics stream."

The "problem stream" is the process by which problems are identified as important to remedy through governmental action. The most significant actors in the process of problem identification and definition are "visible" actors such as legislators, cabinet members, and executives (e.g., the president). There are several ways that problems can gain attention. These include "indicators," which are routine data collected and analyzed by governmental and nongovernmental policy actors; ongoing "feedback" about the operation of existing programs; and "focusing events." Examples of focusing events are a bridge collapse, a plane crash, or long lines at gas stations during an oil shortage. Often groups that have been trying to focus attention on a problem (or a solution) can take advantage of the interest that the media, the general public, and policymakers give to such a "crisis."

The "policy stream" consists of the interaction and recombination of policy ideas, some of which emerge as viable and some of which do not survive, within a specific policy arena. The creation, exchange, and evaluation of these ideas are conducted by the members of the "policy community," specialists in a given policy area who interact with one another from various institutional positions in and outside of government. These specialists can be staff of Congress, executive branch agencies or interest groups, academics, or employees of independent policy organizations or "think tanks." The third stream, the "politics stream," describes the characteristics of the nation's politics at a particular point in time, including which parties or factions within parties control the White House and Congress.

Kingdon argues that a subject is most likely to rise on the decision agenda when these three separate streams—problems, policies, and politics—come together. When this happens, a "window of opportunity" opens for action on a given problem. Such an opportunity may be seized by "policy entrepreneurs"—those individuals *inside or outside* of government who are willing to invest resources such as energy, money, time, and reputation to achieve a particular policy outcome.

Policy entrepreneurs play a central role in Kingdon's theory about how subjects get on the governmental agenda. They work to get recognition for a problem, defining it in the way that will be most effective. They are persistent in putting forward new ideas both within the policy community and outside of it, including introducing bills, holding hearings, giving speeches, and issuing studies and reports—a process that Kingdon calls "softening up." After the softening up process, successful entrepreneurs may be able to use an opportunity in the problem stream (interest by powerful actors) or a shift in the political stream (e.g., a new administration) to integrate problems, proposals, and politics.

Following Kingdon, policy developments in child health are conceptualized as the interaction of the activities of entrepreneurs within a policy network supportive of expansions of health-care access with changes in the larger political environment. In the case of children's health insurance, activity within the policy community and significant events in Kingdon's "political stream" explain agenda-building and policy formulation. Over time, children's advocates have both responded to and attempted to influence the broader policy agenda.

In Chapter 2, I describe the emergence of a child health policy community during the 1980s that shared a set of beliefs about the nature of appropriate child health services and the necessity for providing them to large numbers of uninsured and underserved children. Several of the institutions within this policy network engaged in activities that aimed to diffuse these beliefs to political actors outside the policy community—that is, to other policymakers and to the general public. There were several policy entrepreneurs whose activities were critical to this effort, including the Children's Defense Fund (CDF) founder Marian Wright Edelman, Governor Richard W. Riley of South Carolina, Congressman George E. Miller (D-CA), and Senator Lawton Chiles (D-FL). One consequence of this focus on children was the expansion of Medicaid eligibility for pregnant women and children and other changes in Medicaid that resulted in an increase in coverage for these populations. Key policy entrepreneurs in that effort were Sara Rosenbaum, the Health Policy Director of CDF; Congressman Henry Waxman (D-CA); and Senator Lloyd Bentsen (D-TX).

In Chapter 3, I chronicle the way in which events in the policy stream interacted with those within the political stream to create the State Children's Health Insurance Program in 1997. While children's health advocates had proposed expansions of insurance coverage for children *before* the introduction of President Clinton's plan for health system "reform" in September 1993, it was the failure of Congress to enact the Clinton plan that provided the impetus for Democratic legislative leaders to move children's health insurance higher on their domestic agenda. Policy entrepreneurs were again critical in the actual enactment of a children's health insurance program. The political dynamic that moved a children's health insurance program through the legislative process was the entrepreneurial activity,[3] in both policy and political terms (Peterson 1993), of two highly respected senators, Edward Kennedy (D-MA) and Orrin Hatch (R-UT), in partnership with CDF, the "premier" children's advocacy group on the national scene.

Kingdon notes that program reauthorization is a time when the policy "window" routinely opens (1995). The SCHIP reauthorization process, which began in 2006, was used by different policy communities to move their specific issues higher on the policy agenda. (Another metaphor for these policy communities and the "window of opportunity" is the theater. The policy agenda is the stage; policy communities work on a multitude of issues "offstage" while preparing for their time "onstage.") These policy communities included those concerned about expanding health coverage for pregnant women, coverage for legal immigrants, and increasing access to dental care for low-income children. The reauthorization of SCHIP did not occur until 2009, after a shift in the political stream. Although reauthorization and expansion had broad support across a coalition of professional and business groups as well as the support of a majority of members of Congress, the program was not reauthorized until there was a new president.

While immensely useful as a general framework for organizing information about the policy process, Kingdon's model needs to be integrated with other conceptual frameworks. The work of Mark Peterson focuses on another critical dimension of policymaking: the ways in which prior policy events influence policymaking at later points in time.

Policy Legacies

Building on the work of Paul Pierson (1992 and see Pierson 2000) and others, Peterson argues that analyzing policy decisions and outcomes only in terms of actors and power arrangements at one point in time is not sufficient to understand the personal, ideological, and institutional dynamics of the event. Rather, it is necessary to examine how prior policy events have shaped the political environment. These policy legacies are "created by previous policy debate, action, and implementation" (Peterson 1997: 1080).

Peterson describes the way that policy legacies enter the policy process via "social learning" by policy actors. He identifies two kinds of social learning, "substantive learning" and "situational learning." Substantive learning is about the policy itself: it "incorporates the results of practice, experimentation, observation, analysis . . . argued on the basis of facts" (1997: 1087). (Although, as he points out—citing Deborah Stone's classic *Policy Paradox* [2012]—there is no actual objective policy analysis because all "facts" are shaped by the ideological prism of the analyst.)

Situational learning, in contrast, involves lessons about which policies are viable in a specific political environment. Different types of policy actors ("experts," "organized interests," "politicians") will differ in the degree to which they use each of these types of learning. Whether substantive or situational learning will be viewed as most important in a specific policy situation is also related to the "scope of the policy," from policy implementation by bureaucrats (more substantive) to the formulation of legislation that could involve major structural change (more situational).

The policy legacies that shaped the enactment and structure of SCHIP included substantive learning about the unique characteristics of children's health and health services, the increasing numbers of uninsured children, and prior state attempts to deal with this problem. SCHIP policy entrepreneurs acted on the basis of situational learning about politically viable health policy proposals in the period after the failure of the Clinton plan for health-care reform and the 1994 election. There were two sets of policy legacies here, one about the failure of universal health insurance and another about conflict related to state versus federal power within the Medicaid program.

While several distinct policy legacies influenced the timing and structure of SCHIP in 1997, the debate over SCHIP reauthorization in 2007 featured the phenomenon of "policy foreshadowing." President Bush and some conservative members of Congress opposed SCHIP reauthorization because they believed that expanding coverage to children in higher-income families would breach a boundary between the public and private health sectors and negatively influence the outcome of future health policy decisions for the entire US population.

Policy Communities: "Advocacy Coalitions"

Kingdon notes that the degree of cohesion or fragmentation of policy communities varies (Kingdon 1995: 118). However, he is not specific about the internal structure of such communities or their boundaries. Paul A. Sabatier's model (1988) of the internal structures of policy communities or subsystems incorporates the effect of specialization, professionalization, and the increased use of policy research in US (particularly federal) policymaking during the past several decades (see Peterson 1995).

Sabatier posits a concept of "advocacy coalitions" whose interactions within various policy domains helps to explain policy change. These advocacy coalitions are defined as networks of individuals from different institutional positions both in and outside of government "who share a particular belief system—i.e., a set of basic values, causal assumptions, and problem perceptions—and who show a non-trivial degree of coordinated activity over time" (Sabatier 1988: 139). The "core" of the belief systems of members of such coalitions include "deep core" assumptions about the nature of human society, notions about justice, priorities of various values, and so on. The next level of beliefs, "the near core," is more concrete and includes such values as the role of the market versus that of government in a particular policy area, and the distribution of authority among levels of government. Advocacy coalitions seek to realize their policy goals by controlling political resources (governmental agencies may be a part of advocacy coalitions) and through debate about policy ideas with representatives of other coalitions. In any specific policy area during the period studied, there may be competing advocacy coalitions with very different core belief systems or there may be one dominant advocacy coalition and one or several minority coalitions. The dominant coalition may be fragmented at various junctures (Sabatier 1988: 142–148).

In the years since Sabatier first developed the advocacy coalition concept, numerous case studies have applied it and suggested refinements and Sabatier and his colleagues have discussed these refinements (Sabatier and Jenkins-Smith 1999; Sabatier and Weible 2007). While such discussions have clarified the necessity of clearly delineating the boundaries of the policy subsystems and studying them over time (seven to ten years is suggested), the core notion of analyzing the interaction of policy actors with shared belief systems is a useful one. The policy network concerned with children's health insurance can be delineated, and I trace its emergence, existence, and internal conflicts for more than twenty years.

Most policy communities in the United States include interest groups whose constituents (large corporations, small businesses, teachers, the elderly) have political resources—money, expertise, numbers and votes, along with organizational and research skills. Potential constituencies with few political resources often remain underrepresented in the policy process. Children—or at least preadolescent children—do not have any political resources. Gilbert Steiner, who examined children's advocacy in the 1970s, rather acidly said, "As political actors children are useless and dependent" (Steiner 1976: 143). Thus the policy community concerned about children's health will consist of groups representing children, rather than children themselves.[4] One would also expect the child health policy community or communities to be less stable than most policy communities, precisely because children themselves lack political resources.

Within the child health policy community there was one dominant advocacy coalition that worked on increasing access to care through insurance coverage and then a competing advocacy coalition that was influential in shaping policy related to the *delivery of child health services* rather than children's health insurance. But there were also some changes in the composition of the dominant advocacy coalition over time and internal conflict over the structure of the State Children's Health Insurance Program. These will be described in Chapters 2 and 3.

It is precisely because children are "resource-less" that both outside groups and inside supportive policymakers must use wise "framing" strategies to build support for the allocation of actual (as opposed to symbolic) benefits for children. An analysis of how children's health issues were framed is thus critical to understanding the nature of the policy process in relation to children's health insurance.

"Framing" Health Insurance for Children

Political scientists have long written about the presentation of policy arguments in a manner that evokes specific values and societal beliefs (Stone [1988] 2012) and about the process by which certain policy ideas are "organized out" of political discourse by being labeled as outside of the US ideological spectrum (Schattschneider 1960; Bachrach and Baratz 1970; Cobb and Elder 1983; Rochefort and Cobb 1994; Cobb and Ross 1997). "Framing" refers to the specific way that political actors present an issue or a policy to an audience, often attempting to link the policy or issue to deeply held common values. Framing is a process of "value recruitment," "efforts of political persuaders to influence the connections individuals make between broad social values and particular political issues" (Nelson, Wittmer, and Shortle 2010: 13). Thus, the works of Schattschneider, Stone, Cobb and Elder, Cobb and Ross, and Bachrach and Baratz are all expositions on framing broadly defined.[5]

Recent political science scholarship that analyzes framing explores the effects of framing on public opinion, often by doing laboratory experiments looking at the impact of various framing strategies on different audiences. It seeks to understand the conditions that make presenting an issue, policy, or event in a certain way more or less effective in shaping public opinion. These are "framing effects" (see Nelson, Wittmer, and Shortle 2010; Gormley 2010). While most of this research examines how the frames created by elected officials and the media are received by the public, there has been some work on how interest groups create frames (Chong and Druckman 2007).

It can be suggested that within a policy network, one set of policy actors uses frames to influence the views, and possibly the behavior, of other elite actors. Members of Congress and their staffs frame issues for each other, and interest groups certainly attempt to frame their arguments in a way that will make members of Congress or agency officials sympathetic to their cause. The goal here was to understand how children's health insurance was framed within the "elite discourse" over time.

In this book, I discuss the framing of the expansion of Medicaid eligibility for pregnant women and children in the 1980s, the framing of the children's health insurance bill proposed by senators Kennedy and Hatch in 1997, and the way that both supporters and opponents framed the expansion and reauthorization of SCHIP in 2007. I show that the frames used by advocates of expanding Medicaid eligibility in the 1980s functioned as a form of "substantive policy learning" and were used again during the debates over both the creation and reauthorization of SCHIP.

Framing in the political debate over the reauthorization of children's health insurance was "emphasis framing" in which "competing frames emphasize different messages" about what is at stake in the policy debate (Schaffner and Sellers 2010). Supporters of expanding the program emphasized the long-term economic value of providing health insurance coverage to large numbers of children, while opponents of expansion—such as the Bush administration—countered with the concept of an expanded SCHIP as a "Trojan horse" ushering in the demise of the "free-market" aspects of the US health-care system.

Schneider and Ingram (1993) discuss one aspect of the embedded historical framing of different kinds of groups over time, the "social construction of target populations." Both the power of specific types of groups and the way that they are constructed and viewed are important in agenda setting and policy outcomes. Children, along with mothers, are in Schneider and Ingram's matrix "dependent groups"—positively constructed but politically weak. Such "dependent groups" may be offered symbolic policies that express concern but do not allocate resources (Schneider and Ingram 1993).

Children are positively constructed within US political culture because of both their vulnerability and their "innocence." In fact, David S. Gutterman argues that *children represent innocence* and shows that the rhetorical response to the 9/11 attacks often used children as a representation of the innocence of the whole nation (Gutterman 2002). Children are innocent in two important ways. First, they are malleable, as adults may not be. They are, in a sense, a "new frontier" where we as a society can begin again and succeed in solving our social problems. "It's easier to build successful children than repair men and women," said the governor of Kentucky and cochair of a National Governors Association (NGA) campaign on children's issues in 1986. Second, children are "innocent" because they have not made the choice to do things that the mainstream culture would consider antisocial—for example, taking illegal drugs or receiving public assistance. (The framing of children as both innocent and dependent on parental decisionmaking is the basis of "The Dream Act," which would have legalized the status of young adults brought to the United States as children by immigrant parents who were undocumented or outstayed their visas.) Even among those with an individualistic view of the origins of poverty and drug addiction, children can be seen as the innocent victims of the actions of adults.

Americans are and have been relatively comfortable supporting government-funded programs for children. A report done for the Democratic Party in 1987 found far more support for social and economic programs that benefited children than for those that assisted adults (Dionne 1987). Public opinion polls conducted between 1990 and 1995 found that majorities of respondents across demographic groups and ideological positions believed that children's health should be prioritized as a government effort. Polls conducted by First Focus in 2010 and 2011 found that large majorities of voters chose children's coverage as their priority for health coverage reform and children's programs as those most important to be protected from federal budget cuts.

Schneider and Ingram also relate the different social constructions of target populations to differing policy rationales. The rationales for policy aimed at powerful, positively constructed groups discuss how fulfilling the needs of those groups will serve important public purposes such as national defense and economic competitiveness, whereas policies benefiting powerless groups are more likely to be justified using social justice–oriented rationales. During the 1980s and 1990s, appeals to social justice and morality were central in the rhetoric of Marian Wright Edelman, the founder of the Children's Defense Fund (CDF). Edelman and CDF, the oldest and most prominent children's advocacy organization, framed their appeals on behalf of public policies that would benefit children in religious and moral language that emphasized children's vulnerability (Marlow 1995). But interestingly, much of the framing used in arguing for the expansion of children's health insurance from the mid-1980s through 2009 was about the economic benefits that such a policy would produce. (CDF used this framing as well.) Such "economic" framing will be discussed at several points in my analysis of the framing of children's health insurance coverage in Chapters 2, 3, and 5.

Framing issues to evoke broadly shared US values was crucial to effective policy advocacy for children's health insurance. These values included the innocence of children, but also positive norms about work and family responsibility and negative values attached to cigarette manufacturers and smoking by youth. Ideological arguments about the boundaries of public health financing were also central to policy debates about children's health insurance because this issue was intertwined with the larger debate about universal health insurance coverage.

The Interview Process

This analysis is based on data from both archival material and interviews with policy actors. Archival data include newspaper and journal accounts, reports published by government agencies and nongovernmental organizations, congressional documents, and congressional office files. I have drawn on data from four different sets of interviews conducted at different points in time.

The first was a set of informant interviews with policy staff at several children's advocacy organizations conducted in the mid-1990s for a project describing the (then) child health policy community; the second was a series of interviews about the agenda-setting process for children's issues in the mid-1980s and the related legislative expansions of Medicaid eligibility for pregnant women and children during the latter part of that decade. The third and fourth sets of interviews were about the policy processes that resulted in the creation of SCHIP in 1997 and the debate over its reauthorization and expansion in 2006–2009, respectively. Those interviewed were participants in some aspect of the policy process that I was investigating: administration officials, staff of public commissions, congressional committees, or interest groups. In several cases I interviewed different staff members working for the same congressional committee or the same not-for-profit organization (such as the American Academy of Pediatrics) at different points in time.[6]

A snowball sampling technique was used to assure that I had identified all of the key participants in each phase of each policy process. I began with a list of participants involved with each of these legislative events, based on archival material and a set of key informant interviews. I asked each interviewee at the end of each meeting who else they believed I should interview. After a certain number of interviews, I found the same names were being suggested by all of the interviewees. This was a confirmation of the policy community or policy network concept.

The interviews that I conducted were semistructured, with open-ended questions. I used two interview tools or questionnaires for each person interviewed. One was a general set of questions about the policy process that we were discussing; a second questionnaire was about the specific role of their organization, institution, or member of Congress in this process. Often those interviewed used the questions as a guide to telling her/his "own story" and sharing insight into the policy process.

All interviews were conducted in confidentiality, and all but two were tape-recorded with the permission of those interviewed. The questions were submitted to those interviewed in advance of our meeting. I informed all interviewees that I would use their institutional positions, rather than their names, in referencing them, and they agreed to this. The institutional positions that are identified are the positions that those interviewed occupied during the policy process that they were discussing and were not necessarily those occupied at the time that the interview took place. Congressional staff are identified by the part of Congress (House or Senate) and the political party of the member of Congress for whom they were working during the period that they were discussing with me, and by a number (Republican Senate staff #3; Democratic House staff #2). Since I conducted interviews with staff of some interest groups more than once, I have also assigned numbers to identify different staff members working for the same group (CDF staff #3). Although all of those who worked for interest groups are identified as "staff," some people had high-level positions in the organizations such as vice president for policy or policy director.

A brief note here about the abbreviations used in this book to refer to the children's health insurance program: The State Children's Health Insurance Program was created by federal legislation in August 1997. Twelve years later it was reauthorized by the Children's Health Insurance Program Reauthorization Act of 2009. Prior to February 4, 2009, when this legislation was signed, the federal children's health insurance program was usually referred to as SCHIP. Since reauthorization, it has been referred to as CHIP. I will use both SCHIP and CHIP, depending on whether I am discussing program and/or policy activity before or after February 2009.[7]

Boundary-Setting:
The History of Federal Child Health Policy

The second part of this chapter will place the emergence of a policy community focused on the expansion of health care for children in the mid-1980s within a larger historical and ideological context. It will outline the politics of federal funding for maternal and child health programs from the early twentieth century through the 1970s.

From the Progressive Era, federally funded child health services were community-based and limited to preventive services such as immunization, parental education, and professional training, and to treatment for a few specified conditions. Children's health advocates, including public health physicians, faced opposition from private providers to public services that would compete with private medicine.

Child Health Advocacy in the Progressive Era

One of the issues addressed by the social reformers of the Progressive period was the welfare of children, particularly poor children.[8] Industrialization, migration, immigration, and urbanization produced high rates of infectious disease and death in infants and young children. Children worked in factories, lived in inadequate housing, and suffered from malnutrition (Black 1988; Wilson 1989). Diarrhea was a major cause of infant death, and one of the first efforts made to reduce infant mortality was the creation of infant milk stations to provide inexpensive sterilized milk in urban working-class areas. In 1908 the New York City Bureau of Child Hygiene was established, the first in the nation. The bureau sent nurses to visit new babies and to teach their mothers how to care for them. It also provided health exams to children in the public schools (Halpern 1988; Wilson 1989). At the national level, activities that focused on child welfare included the first White House conference on children in 1908, the birth of the American Association for the Prevention of Infant Mortality in 1910, and the establishment of the US Children's Bureau in 1912 (Halpern 1988).

Most of the child health activists, in both private organizations and government agencies, were women. The League of Women Voters and the Women's Joint Congressional Committee worked with other activists for the passage of the Maternity and Infancy (Sheppard-Towner) Act of 1921, legislation that provided federal matching funds to states to establish prenatal and child health services. Opponents of the legislation included the American Medical Association (AMA), chiropractors, and those opposed to women's suffrage. During the debate, members of Congress made antifeminist remarks and the AMA labeled the act as "socialistic." Women's magazines were very supportive of the legislation, and the potential votes of newly enfranchised women were a major factor in its passage (Black 1988; Wilson 1989).

The Sheppard-Towner Act was the first federal grant-in-aid program in health care. Sheppard-Towner funds were used to establish 3,000 clinics where women physicians and public health nurses examined children and taught their mothers and older sisters (in "little mothers" classes) about infant care, nutrition, and childhood illness (Black 1988). The renewal of Sheppard-Towner (five years after enactment) was actively opposed by the AMA and the Catholic Church. Congress voted to extend the legislation for two years and then to repeal it (Wilson 1989).

Two aspects of child health advocacy in the first part of the twentieth century are noteworthy. First, women physicians who established maternal and child health programs incorporated the values of the female-dominated popular health movement of the nineteenth century by emphasizing the education of mothers, preventive services such as immunization and nutrition counseling, and work in the community, such as "family visitors."

Second, these health activists avoided direct competition with general practitioners by not providing treatment for illness (Black 1988). This was part of the general struggle between public health and academic physicians and private-practice physicians over the boundaries of public and private medicine during the late nineteenth and early twentieth centuries. This "boundary-setting" also involved means testing, such as was imposed on urban dispensaries in New York State in 1899 (Sardell 1988: ch. 2). The belief that publicly funded medical care should only be provided to the very poor—those proven not to be able to pay for their care—was echoed in the debate over the expansion of SCHIP in 2007, particularly in the discussion of "crowd-out" (the substitution of public coverage for private insurance).

Pediatrics and the Child Welfare Movement

Pediatricians had a special relationship to the child health movement, which was quite different from that of most general practitioners and the AMA. Pediatrics began to develop as a specialty during the second half of the nineteenth century, primarily as a separate academic area.[9] In contrast to other medical specialties, pediatrics defined itself as providing preventive and primary care and focusing on normal development rather than pathology. Pediatricians worked in the child welfare movement, providing it with greater legitimacy and using it to support their demands for the recognition of pediatrics as a unique medical specialty (see Halpern 1988). Yet by the 1930s, the majority of pediatricians were in private practice, providing services primarily to children in middle-class families.

The child health clinics established in the 1920s offered "well-baby conferences" during which health professionals evaluated children's development and advised mothers on many aspects of child rearing. Such services were promoted by the Children's Bureau and national child health organizations, and a demand for them was generated among middle-class as well as working-class mothers. In response, one group of pediatricians campaigned to restrict the use of clinics to families unable to pay for private pediatric care (Halpern 1988). A specialty that was nurtured by a social movement to improve the health of poor mothers and children was privatized.[10]

The Depression and World War II

The Sheppard-Towner Act expired just as the Depression began, and states were unable to provide maternal and child health care (Wilson 1989). While proposals for universal health insurance were excluded from the Roosevelt administration's draft of the Social Security bill because of the opposition of the AMA (Stevens 1971: 188, 190), Sheppard-Towner was reborn as Title V of the Social Security Act of 1935. Title V was to be administered by the Children's Bureau[11] and included funds for maternal and child health services and for identifying and treating conditions that could result in crippling.

Until the beginning of World War II, Title V primarily funded programs for planning, training, and preventive health projects. Little direct medical care was provided, again in observation of the boundaries between public and private medicine. However, during World War II, the Children's Bureau administered a separate program of prenatal and obstetrical care for the wives of servicemen, the Emergency Maternity and Infant Care Program. This was the largest tax-supported medical care program ever funded solely by the federal government (Wilson 1989). Opposition to the expansion of publicly funded medical care was deflected by labeling it as an emergency program and by limiting it to the wives of servicemen in the lowest pay grades. One and a half million women received care under the Emergency Maternity and Infant Care Program, and although maternal and child health programs were again limited to preventive health services after 1949, a precedent had been established for providing federally funded prenatal, obstetrical, and postpartum care (Davis and Schoen 1978; Marieskind 1980).

The Expansion of Child Health Services During the 1960s

During the 1960s, when the role of the federal government in social policy was broadened, low-income women and children became the beneficiaries of more extensive health-care financing and services. In 1965, Medicaid was enacted along with Medicare. Medicaid provided federal funds to the states on a cost-sharing basis to pay for medical services to the poor, primarily provided by the private sector. Medicaid became the major source of public funding for children's health services.

As early as 1966, the Department of Health, Education, and Welfare (DHEW) proposed that state Medicaid agencies take direct responsibility for the provision of preventive health services to low-income families, a responsibility not being fulfilled by private practitioners. This proposal became the Early Periodic Screening, Diagnosis, and Treatment (EPSDT) program enacted by Congress as part of the Social Security Amendments of 1967. States were required to screen all Medicaid-eligible children for potentially handicapping conditions and then to arrange treatment. Advocates for the EPSDT program hoped that the program would be structured to bring together all children's health services (Goggin 1987), but this was not done.

In 1965, as part of the War on Poverty, the federal government funded a small demonstration project to establish neighborhood health centers with the goal of increasing access to health care and providing a model of comprehensive, community-oriented care. In 1975, these programs received their own separate legislative authority as community health centers (CHCs), but in the same year DHEW shifted funding from a small number of comprehensive centers based on a social medicine model to a larger number of more traditional medical projects. The number of community health centers in medically underserved areas was increased during the Carter administration, and later greatly expanded by both the administration of George W. Bush and the first Obama administration. Most of those served by CHCs are women and children (Sardell 1988, 2012). Also during the 1960s, Congress created a program to fund family planning services and the Women, Infants, and Children program (WIC), which provided nutritious food and nutrition counseling to pregnant and lactating women and children up to age five. Studies indicated that these programs successfully increased access to care for low-income pregnant women and children and helped to reduce mortality and morbidity among children (Starfield 1985).

Retrenchment in Federal Spending for Maternal and Child Services

While the first ten years of the Medicaid program saw expansion in eligibility and benefits, the second decade was, particularly for children's health services, a period of retrenchment. During the latter part of the 1970s, inflation rates were almost as high as increases in program expenditures, so the actual availability of services expanded only slightly. Beginning in 1972, there was a shift within Medicaid away from spending on health services for nondisabled children as a higher proportion of Medicaid funds went to pay for services for the aged, blind, and disabled. In 1972, 18 percent of all Medicaid expenditures paid for services for nondisabled children under 21; in 1987, the proportion was 13 percent (Oberg and Polich 1988).

In the early part of the 1980s, both Medicaid funding and funding for federal grant programs in maternal and child health were cut as part of the Reagan administration's efforts to cut spending on domestic social programs. These cuts threatened the gains made in maternal and child health and stimulated a new focus on children's issues during the 1980s. New children's health advocates emerged, and new policy arguments were made about the morality and cost-effectiveness of the expansion of government funding for children's health services. These events are described in Chapter 2.

Notes

1. This has changed as the intense ideological polarization in Washington has made other program reauthorizations controversial. A case in point is the conflict over the reauthorization of the Violence Against Women Act, another program whose targets—physically and sexually abused individuals—would appear to be universally sympathetic. (See Weisman 2013.)

2. In their books, David Smith, Laura Olson, and Frank Thompson also discuss the enactment and implementation of SCHIP.

3. Oliver and Paul-Shaheen (1997) use their empirical work on comprehensive health-care reform in the states to illustrate a model of policy entrepreneurship that conceptualizes the set of activities in which successful policy entrepreneurs engage as parallel to those of entrepreneurs in a corporate environment. Thus, recruiting others from in or outside of government to work with them as "investors" is necessary, as is gathering broader support from policymakers, interest groups, or the interested public by framing the issue in ways that will attract support ("marketing").

4. Historically, such groups have been linked to other reform movements, such as the Progressive movement and the women's movement (Skocpol 1992; Imig 2001).

5. In part because scholarly work on this concept is done from several different disciplines including sociology, mass communication, and political science, there is no agreement on a general definition of framing (Schaffner and Sellers 2010).

6. I conducted twenty-seven interviews (between October 1998 and June 1999) with policy actors who participated in or observed the creation of SCHIP: sixteen Senate and House committee staff, ten interest group officials or staff, and one member of the Clinton White House staff. Between November 2000 and August 2001, I did twenty interviews—seven with congressional staff members, three with staff of government commissions, and ten with officials and staff of interest group or advocacy organizations—about efforts to expand Medicaid eligibility to pregnant women and children. (Three of these were phone interviews and were conducted jointly with Kay A. Johnson, the co-investigator of a project analyzing several different child health policy issues, and funded by the Robert Wood Johnson Foundation Investigator Award in Health Policy Research from 1999 to 2003). In October and December 2010, I interviewed three Senate staff members and the staff of five interest or advocacy organizations active on the issue of reauthorizing SCHIP. All of the in-person interviews were conducted in Washington, DC.

7. States have their own names for the children's health insurance programs that receive funding through the federal program: for example, Dr. Dyna-

sur in Vermont, Husky Health in Connecticut, NewMexikids and NewMexi-Teens in New Mexico.

8. This historical discussion is reproduced from my article, "Child Health Policy in the U.S.: The Paradox of Consensus" (1990) by permission of the *Journal of Health Politics, Policy and Law* in which it appeared. It was updated and appeared in *Health Policy and the Disadvantaged,* edited by Lawrence D. Brown (Durham, NC: Duke University Press, 1991).

9. A section on diseases of children was created by the AMA in 1879; the American Pediatric Society was created in 1888 (Wilson 1989).

10. Pediatricians, however, continued to be active on social policy issues. During the 1930s, (male) pediatricians replaced feminist political activists in policy positions in government and private sector organizations concerned with children's health (Black 1988).

11. The Children's Bureau had originally been located in the Department of Labor, but was transferred to the Federal Security Agency in 1946. That agency became the Department of Health, Education, and Welfare (DHEW) in 1953. In 1967, the Children's Bureau lost most of its programs to other bureaus in DHEW. Title V came under the jurisdiction of the Public Health Service (Wilson 1989). In 1980, DHEW became the Department of Health and Human Services (DHHS) after the creation of the Department of Education in 1979.

2

The Emergence of the Child Health Advocacy Community

During the 1980s, there was a new focus on "children's issues." A child health "policy network" or policy community emerged that shared a set of beliefs about the nature of appropriate child health services and the necessity for providing them to large numbers of uninsured and underserved children. This policy network of both public institutions and private organizations was created during the process of producing and sharing information about the health status of low-income US children. One outcome of the efforts of policy entrepreneurs within this community was a series of Medicaid eligibility expansions during the second half of the 1980s that increased health insurance coverage for pregnant women and children. These expansions were supported by a bipartisan, trans-ideological coalition within Congress that viewed children as particularly worthy of social support for both moral and pragmatic reasons.

In this chapter, I describe the emergence and evolution of this child health policy community, the public and private actors within it, the process of expanding Medicaid eligibility, and the way that the arguments in favor of Medicaid eligibility expansions were framed.

The Emergence of Children's Advocacy

The Baseline

The scholarly work published to date about the private organizations and public institutions advocating for improved health care for children during the 1960s and 1970s is quite limited.¹ Gilbert Y. Steiner did survey the state of policy advocacy for children in the 1970s in his book *The Children's Cause* (1976), and this work can thus be used as a baseline description of the time just before "children's issues" emerged on the policy agenda. Steiner's chapter "Lobbyists for Children" discusses organizations concerned with child development, early childhood education, adoption, and foster care services. His descriptions of federal child health programs and policies during the 1960s and 1970s (he was not explicitly concerned with the concept of policy communities) suggest that a fragmented set of maternal and child health programs funded under Title V of the Social Security Act was supported by equally fragmented and small numbers of advocates for children's health services.²

In general, Steiner found limited interest on the part of congressional or bureaucratic actors in children's health and little advocacy activity on children's issues. He discusses only two national groups active on children's health issues, the "dying National Welfare Rights Organization" concerned about the Early Periodic Screening, Diagnosis, and Treatment (EPSDT) program and the Association of Children and Youth Project Directors fighting to continue their new categorical grants during the Nixon administration (Steiner 1976: ch. 9). He identifies the Children's Defense Fund (CDF) as the most potentially effective advocacy group working on behalf of children, although he is not sure that CDF will survive (Steiner 1976: 175). In fact, CDF became the premier advocate for low-income children on a wide range of issues, including education, child care, income support, housing, and health care. In 1993, CDF was called "the nation's most prominent child advocacy group . . . enjoying unprecedented political influence" by Jason DeParle in the *New York Times* (DeParle 1993).

The CDF and CHAP

CDF's origins are in the experiences that its founder, Marian Wright Edelman, and others of its original senior staff had in the civil rights and antipoverty movements of the 1960s. Edelman was a young civil rights attorney in Mississippi (the first African American woman to pass the bar in that state) and a board member of the Child Development Group of Mississippi, a federally funded antipoverty agency. The agency ran a Head Start program and did community organizing with the families of the children who were enrolled. After witnessing the attacks of white southern US senators on the agency, which almost lost its funding, Edelman decided that she wanted to work to influence the federal policy process in Washington.

Edelman's early work in Washington suggested to her that divisions of class and race might be bridged by placing children's needs at the center of the political discussion. The hope was that innocent and vulnerable children would be viewed as appropriate beneficiaries of societal and governmental support. In 1973 Edelman founded the Children's Defense Fund with support from private foundations. The organization was successful in working to increase funding for Head Start during the Nixon administration, expanding educational opportunities for children with disabilities, establishing the rights of foster children for services, prohibiting housing discrimination against families with children, and expanding tax relief for low-income families. CDF staff did research on the needs of low-income children in the United States, brought that research to both Congress and the media, developed legislative strategies, and coordinated the work of state and local organizations focusing on these needs. By the 1990s, CDF had field offices in nine states and an extensive network of faith-based communities (Sardell 1995).

Marian Wright Edelman and CDF framed the necessity to act in moral terms. Edelman is an eloquent, charismatic speaker in the tradition of the African American church, and she captured the attention of the media during the 1980s and 1990s by framing discussions of education, income, health, and juvenile justice policy in terms of the moral responsibility that US society had for its children. She combined a "liberal" "language of rights" with a religiously based "language of good" in her appeals for support of children's needs. As discussions of morality in social policy, framed in religious terms by the Right, became more central in US political debates, Edelman was said to be the singular representative of the use of religiously based moral rhetoric on the Left (Marlow 1995).[3]

Through its research, publications, and outreach to the media, as well as Edelman's charismatic rhetorical style, CDF had a critical role in creating a national dialogue on children's issues (Tompkins 1989; Marlow 1995). This critical role can be measured very concretely by noting that its logo, used extensively in what would be called "branding" today, is "Leave No Child Behind." In the 2000 presidential election, the Republican candidates circulated a button that said "No Child Left Behind—Bush Cheney 2000." And this became the name of the Bush administration's educational "reform" initiative that was enacted in 2001.

Sara Rosenbaum and Kay A. Johnson, staff members in CDF's Health Division, were the outside policy entrepreneurs who were key to the enactment of the expansion of Medicaid eligibility for low-income women and children during the 1980s. They worked with members of Congress and their staffs and created a coalition of supportive outside organizations.

In the late 1970s, right after the publication of Steiner's work, advocates both inside and outside the Carter administration made an effort to convince Congress to expand eligibility and services for pregnant women and children within the Medicaid program. President Jimmy Carter initially proposed using Medicaid expansion as a vehicle for covering all of the uninsured, but when the universal plan became politically infeasible, attention shifted to expanding Medicaid coverage for children. However, efforts in both the 95th and 96th Congresses (1977–1980) to get congressional approval of the administration's Child Health Assessment Program (CHAP) failed. One reason was that members of the House attached antiabortion amendments to the Medicaid expansion legislation (Rosenbaum and Sonosky 2001: fn. 3). Others were the failure of child advocates to work together to educate lawmakers and the media on the issues and the lack of congressional proponents. However, by 1984, when a similar effort was successful, many of these barriers had been overcome (Johnson, Hughes, and Rosenbaum 1988). By the mid-1980s, the media was discussing a "crisis" in child health, CDF had organized a coalition of supportive organizations, and members of Congress such as congressmen George Miller and Henry Waxman and senators Lawton Chiles and Lloyd Bentsen were acting as policy entrepreneurs: Miller on "children's issues" in general, Chiles on infant mortality, and Waxman and Bentsen on Medicaid. The impetus for renewed policy activity related to children's issues *in general* were the policy decisions of the Reagan administration in the early1980s.

Entrepreneurship on "Children's Issues"

Medicaid funding and funding for other federal health programs were cut as part of the Reagan administration's efforts to reduce spending for social programs and to return fiscal and administrative responsibility to the states. In addition, categorical grant programs for children's health and other services were replaced by block grants to the states, which were funded at lower levels than the total funding for the categorical programs. These reductions in funding for maternal and child health and nutrition programs came as economic conditions were worsening and unemployment was increasing. Stories about poverty among pregnant women and sick and malnourished children were reported in the media (Rosenbaum 1988). New children's advocacy groups were created, and advocates from different policy arenas began to work together. There was a surge of activity on behalf of low-income children at the local, state, and national levels. CDF and other groups published detailed reports on both the state of children's welfare and spending on children's programs. During this period of the early to mid 1980s, the activity of both private advocacy groups and public institutions began to focus the attention of policymakers and the media on children's issues. Several new *public institutions* concerned with the needs of children were created during the 1980s.

The House Select Committee on Children, Youth, and Families. The thirty-member House Select Committee on Children, Youth, and Families began work in March 1983 and was disbanded ten years later. The February 1983 vote to establish the select committee was a result of years of entrepreneurial activity by Congressman George Miller (who became its chairman), media attention to the impact of the cuts in social programs, the recognition of women as voters concerned about these issues, and the mobilization of a policy community of advocacy groups focused on children and families.[4] Its purpose was to examine data and explore issues related to the status of children and families (Roberts 1983) and to consciously engage members across the ideological spectrum with these issues. According to a longtime senior staff member of the select committee, "the fact that members of the Committee really did span the most liberal members of Congress to the most conservative members of Congress was valuable. We wanted to get everyone in the same tent if we could."[5] The staff of the committee helped to build consensus around policy ideas like the importance of prevention by presenting the testimony of academic researchers and then arranging for members to gain experiential knowledge by visiting neonatal units, homeless shelters, and day-care programs at field hearings in different parts of the country.[6] For example, a series of field hearings was held about the relationship between low birth weight and access to prenatal care. (The committee held more than eighty hearings during its tenure.) The work of the select committee influenced several conservative members of the House to support the expansion of Medicaid eligibility for low-income pregnant women and children (Kosterlitz 1986b).

The Southern Regional Task Force on Infant Mortality. The Southern Regional Task Force on Infant Mortality was established in 1984 as a joint project of the Southern Legislative Conference and the Southern Governors' Association. Its members included academic and government experts in maternal and child health, religious and civil rights leaders, child advocacy organizations (both CDF and March of Dimes officials were members), and elected officials from all levels of government (Southern Regional Task Force on Infant Mortality 1985). Nine of the eleven states with the highest infant mortality in the United States were southern states; the goals of the task force were to bring attention to the problem and develop policy recommendations to improve maternal and infant health in the region (Williams and Harrison-Clark 1989). The task force held hearings all over the south and issued several reports on their research findings. Its work helped to gain support from southern Republican members of Congress for the expansion of Medicaid eligibility.[7]

One of the task force's recommendations was to allow states to include all pregnant women and children in families with incomes below the poverty level in their Medicaid programs, regardless of employment status or family structure. This would mean expanding Medicaid eligibility beyond the population receiving public assistance. The Southern Governors' Association adopted this recommendation, and the chair of its task force on infant mortality, Governor Richard W. Riley of South Carolina, was a key policy entrepreneur in fostering its adoption by the National Governors Association (Williams and Harrison-Clark 1989).[8] The NGA endorsement was, according to a staff member of the task force, "unusual" because of its cost to the states. Riley also personally visited key members of Congress in support of Medicaid eligibility expansions, and was successful in getting their support, including that of conservative Senator Strom Thurmond (Kosterlitz 1986b).

The National Commission to Prevent Infant Mortality. The National Commission to Prevent Infant Mortality was created by Congress in 1986 to analyze public policies related to the health of infants and women of reproductive age. Its members included representatives of state government, health professionals, members of Congress, and Reagan administration officials. As in the case of the House Select Committee on Children, Youth, and Families, its creation was the result of entrepreneurial activity by a member of Congress, Senator Lawton

Chiles of Florida (Barone and Ujifusa 1986: 238). Chiles became interested in this issue through a personal experience—one of his grandchildren was born prematurely and almost did not survive.

The national commission, along with the Congressional Office of Technology Assessment (OTA) and private organizations such as the Ford Foundation and the Committee for Economic Development (a research organization funded by Fortune 500 corporations) issued reports during the latter part of the 1980s that included policy recommendations to improve the health status of US children. All of these reports agreed on the need for comprehensive, integrated, community-based health, education, and social services for pregnant women and children and shared the assumption that government should assure that these services were provided. These public institutions and private organizations were part of the broad child health "dominant advocacy coalition" that emerged during the 1980s. Within this advocacy coalition were also the interest group staffs and members of Congress and their staffs who worked together to expand Medicaid eligibility for low-income pregnant women and children.

Medicaid Expansion and the Child Health Advocacy Coalition

The Expansion of Medicaid Eligibility

In 1984, provisions included in the Deficit Reduction Act "decoupled" Medicaid from Aid to Families with Dependent Children (AFDC) by requiring eligibility for Medicaid to be based on family income without regard to family structure. This meant that low-income pregnant women and children in families not receiving public assistance could qualify for Medicaid. This was followed by a series of legislative enactments that greatly expanded eligibility levels for pregnant women and children, and restructured the eligibility process itself (see Sardell and Johnson 1998). Expansions in Medicaid eligibility and benefits were enacted as part of the budget reconciliation process in 1985, 1986, 1987, 1989, and 1990. New provisions would first be state options and then later become federal requirements. States were required to establish application sites at community locations separate from Medicaid offices, to provide continuous coverage for pregnant women through the postpartum period and for children to their first birthday, to cover pregnant women and children up to age six with family incomes up to 133 percent of the federal poverty level (FPL), and to provide insurance to children up to age eighteen with family incomes less than 100 percent of the FPL (this last requirement was to be phased in by 2002) (Coughlin, Ku, and Holahan 1994). The significance of these incremental policy changes was to create a federal entitlement for health insurance coverage for children and pregnant women in low-income and "moderate income working families" that was separated from public assistance and the process of applying for public assistance (Rosenbaum and Sonosky 2001).

The Medicaid expansions were initiated by Congressman Henry Waxman (D-CA), who was the chair of the Health Subcommittee of the House Energy and Commerce Committee; Senator Lloyd Bentsen (D-TX), chair of the Senate Finance Committee; and their staffs. The expansions were supported by other committee members and by a coalition of children's advocacy and other groups, led by CDF. From 1984 until 1989 these included the American Academy of Pediatrics, the March of Dimes, the National Association of Community Health Centers,[9] the Association of Maternal and Child Health Programs, the United States Catholic Conference,[10] and the National Governors Association. In Congress there was bipartisan, trans-ideological support for the Medicaid expansions extending from liberal members of Congress like Mickey Leland (D-CA) to Henry Hyde, a conservative Republican from Illinois who sponsored the 1976 amendment that prohibited federal funding of abortions. The support of the Catholic Conference was critical to the support of socially conservative members of Congress, and key to this support was an agreement made by CDF, the Catholic Conference, and key committee staff to separate child health issues from the abortion issue (Rosenbaum 1988).

Congressman Waxman became known as "Mr. Medicaid," a champion of expanding Medicaid to cover poor pregnant women, children, the disabled, and the elderly poor. He used his budgetary expertise and his ability to work across party lines to put the Medicaid expansions within omnibus reconciliation bills that funded many other programs and were therefore less likely to be vetoed (Kosterlitz 1989; Thompson 2012: ch. 3).[11] He was "notorious in reconciliation conferences for tenaciously waiting out his colleagues until he [got] his Medicaid increases" (Rovner 1989: 801). A congressional colleague, George Miller, noted, "You'd get down to the last negotiation with the conferees, and the last question to be asked would be, 'Has Henry signed off?'" (Kosterlitz 1989: 580).

The Core Child Advocacy Groups

Within the broad coalition that supported the Medicaid eligibility expansions was a smaller core group of five organizations that met informally for about ten years to share information and strategize about Medicaid and other federal child health programs. This informal "maternal and child health coalition" was created in 1986 after a disagreement among groups on a proposal for adolescent health programs within Title V. It was chaired by CDF staff. The other groups were the American Academy of Pediatrics (AAP), the Association of Maternal and Child Health Programs (AMCHP), the March of Dimes, and the National Association of Children's Hospitals and Related Institutions (NACHRI). It was an ad hoc coalition with regular meetings but no formal bylaws, formal membership, stationery, or funding. Its membership included additional groups at various points in time. In 1995, two subcommittees of the coalition were formed, one to work on Medicaid issues and the other on budget and appropriations related to children's health programs.[12]

This informal network of interest groups concerned about children's health coverage has continued to function up to the present, although the role of facilitator has moved from CDF to the AAP. Three of these organizations—the AAP, NACHRI, and the March of Dimes—were continually active on the issue of health insurance for pregnant women and children from efforts to expand Medicaid in the 1980s through the reauthorization of SCHIP in 2009. AMCHP, an association of state maternal and child health officials who oversee Title V (maternal and child health) programs, was a key member of the informal maternal and child coalition but not a central actor on SCHIP. CDF, the major nongovernmental or "outside" policy entrepreneur on both the Medicaid expansions and the creation of SCHIP, has already been discussed. I will next describe the AAP, NACHRI, and the March of Dimes, as well as Families USA and the National Governors Association (NGA). Families USA was not a policy actor on children's health during the Medicaid expansions but became very active as a supporter of SCHIP and its expansion. The National Governors Association has been a key actor in Medicaid policy since the program's enactment in 1965 (Ramsay 1995c).

The American Academy of Pediatrics. The establishment of the American Academy of Pediatrics in 1930 by a small group of pediatricians was related both to the development of pediatrics as a specialty within medicine and to a long political conflict over the Sheppard-Towner Act within the American Medical Association (AMA). The AMA's Section on Pediatrics supported it, while the House of Delegates opposed it as "socialistic." Since its formation (and incorporation in Illinois), the AAP has functioned as a traditional professional association, recognizing subspecialties and creating subspecialty boards and conducting educational activities for its members. But after an internal dispute in the 1960s about the organization's presence in the federal policy process, the academy has embraced policy activism. A Washington, DC, office was opened in 1970.

In addition to children's health insurance coverage and access to care—the primary policy concerns of the AAP—the academy works on a broad range of issues that affect children's health and safety, such as tobacco advertising, seat belt and gun regulation, and family and medical leave. The AAP had a membership of about 44,000 in the United States, Canada, and Latin America in 1995 (Ramsay 1995a), and 60,000 in 2013.[13]

It has held an annual legislative conference in Washington since 1987 where its members learn about the legislative process and then meet with their congressional representatives. AAP members are also encouraged to meet with these legislators in their home offices and to invite them to their medical practices. Legislators are particularly receptive to policy-related "stories" told by doctors in the communities that they represent.[14]

The National Association of Children's Hospitals and Related Institutions. The National Association of Children's Hospitals and Related Institutions was founded by twenty-five children's hospitals in 1968 as a not-for-profit charitable organization.[15] In addition to educational activities and research, the association's goals were to develop new financing and delivery systems for children's health care and "to be a visible advocate at both the state and national level for public policy favorable to the well-being of children and the children's hospitals and related institutions which provide their care."[16]

There are three types of institutions that belong to NACHRI: freestanding acute care children's hospitals, smaller rehabilitation or specialty hospitals that serve only chronically ill children, and the pediatric departments of major university medical centers. The missions of these hospitals are clinical care, graduate medical education, biomedical and health services research, and advocacy for children "that may involve issues that don't directly relate to the service delivery of the hospital."[17] These hospitals, in comparison to other hospitals, treat a high proportion of children who receive Medicaid (about 43 percent of revenues) and about 75 percent of the care provided is to children with chronic or congenital conditions. These characteristics are related because children with chronic and/or complex conditions are more likely to be disabled and qualify for Medicaid. In addition, children's hospitals have on-site Medicaid enrollment and an uninsured child who is treated will be screened to see if they are Medicaid eligible. But because insured parents can take their children to any type of health facility, privately insured children treated in children's hospitals tend to have more complex medical conditions, whereas Medicaid-insured children are likely to be receiving a range of services from children's hospitals, including primary and preventive care.

While NACHRI has been involved in a broad range of issues related to children's health and health care—limiting access to guns and tobacco products, seat belt and bicycle helmet requirements, greater funding for graduate medical education and pediatric research, greater accountability of managed care systems—Medicaid and children's health insurance coverage have been the most important issues for the organization over the years.

NACHRI has several different kinds of political resources. First, like the AAP, it is financed by member dues and therefore does not have to expend organizational resources on fundraising and creating a public presence or image in order to get donations. The individual hospital members of NACHRI often have positive public images in their communities and may also have government relations or public relations staffs of their own. Members of hospital boards are often business people and community leaders who may be moderate or conservative politically and can be influential if they speak to conservative or moderate members of Congress. And children's hospitals can present compelling stories to legislators about ill or disabled children and about the economic difficulties of families with children treated at these hospitals. In fact, NACHRI staff noted that there have been several members of Congress whose own children have been treated at children's hospitals and who became their champions, as well as champions of increased Medicaid funding, even when they did not historically support Medicaid. "They just looked through the lens of their own experience—what their child received from this hospital—and now want to enable us to do the same thing for somebody else's child."[18]

The March of Dimes. From the 1980s through the reauthorization of SCHIP in 2009, the March of Dimes was the chief advocate for increased access to health services for pregnant women. The organization was established as the National Foundation for Infantile Paralysis in 1938 to fund research on polio and therapy for its victims; it supported the development of both the Salk and Sabine polio vaccines. It began to work on the issue of birth defects in 1958, and in 1979 it was renamed the March of Dimes Birth Defects Foundation.

The March of Dimes is a national nonprofit volunteer organization with professional staff in both its national headquarters in White Plains, New York, and its Washington, DC, office. It raises funds for research related to birth defects and maternal and infant health more generally. It has advocated on the issues of federal research funding for birth defects, and supported government programs to promote access to maternal and child health, such as immunizations, WIC, and Medicaid (Ramsay 1995b). In 2003, it launched a national campaign against premature births.[19]

The March of Dimes has always been viewed as nonpartisan or bipartisan. It also has a broad volunteer base at the local community level. (In fact, according to a March of Dimes policy official, one-quarter of the freshmen Republican members of Congress in 1994 were or had been volunteers for the March of Dimes.) This has provided opportunities for discussions with a wide range of elected officials on children's health issues. For example, March of Dimes officials and policy staff met with Speaker Newt Gingrich at a testimonial dinner given for him by the Georgia Chapter in 1995 and discussed Medicaid policy. This discussion could probably not have been held with CDF officials.[20]

Families USA. Families USA was established in 1981 as the Villers Foundation with the mission of improving the lives of the elderly poor through legal assistance and policy advocacy. In 1989, it broadened its agenda to include income and health access issues across all age groups and became Families USA. It is a staff rather than a membership group and located in Washington, DC. One of its strategies has been to produce research on policy issues and then to successfully disseminate it to the media. But it also became a leader in working with other groups on "campaign" issues like long-term care, health reform (Oberlander 1995), and SCHIP reauthorization.

The National Governors Association. The NGA, along with other organizations that represent executive and legislative officials from state and local governments, is considered to be part of the "intergovernmental lobby." These groups of public officials engage in all the advocacy strategies that private interest groups do: research, developing relationships with the media, and communicating their views to national policymakers (Cigler 2011). The NGA represents the governors of all the states and five territories and has been a major voice on health-care policy since the 1960s when Medicaid was enacted.

US governors began meeting annually in a Governors' Conference in 1910 and became more interested in influencing national policymaking as the role of the federal government expanded in various domestic policy areas. In 1975, the Governors' Conference became the NGA, a not-for-profit organization with a professional staff, an executive committee, and policy area committees of governors. The executive director of the organization as well as individual governors were frequent witnesses at congressional hearings during the 1980s and 1990s (Ramsay 1995c).

The National Governors Association was an important part of the coalition supporting the initial expansions of Medicaid eligibility for pregnant women and children in the mid-1980s. As noted earlier, this support came through the entrepreneurial efforts of southeastern governors, particularly Governor Richard W. Riley of South Carolina, who was the chair of the Southern Regional Task Force on Infant Mortality. By 1990, however, the NGA was no longer supportive of further Medicaid expansions. One of the reasons was the belief of the governors (particularly Republican governors) that EPSDT was very costly for their states. Not only did the NGA refuse to support further Medicaid expansions, they attempted to end the Medicaid program as a federal "entitlement."

EPSDT, Republican Governors, and Shifts in the Medicaid Expansion Coalition

As noted in Chapter 1, the EPSDT program was created as part of Medicaid in 1967 to guarantee that children were screened and treated for potentially serious health conditions. While this provision is notable as the first federal effort to set standards for comprehensive and preventive health care for a large population, the regulations were not written for three years (Stevens and Stevens 1974). State implementation during the next twenty years was problematic. In response, one provision of the Omnibus Budget Reconciliation Act of 1989 (a large budget package that included incremental Medicaid expansions) explicitly required that states pay for all necessary treatment for conditions found through screening, whether or not the services were included in that state's Medicaid plan. While the effect of this provision on state implementation of EPSDT requirements was limited, governors and other state officials believed that this requirement was a costly one for their states. The EPSDT program became a symbol for many governors of the federal infringement of state autonomy in the form of "unfunded mandates." State officials supported the second set of Medicaid reforms in 1986 and 1987, but by 1990, the state officials— particularly the NGA—resisted further "unfunded mandates" that might drive up state spending.

When the Republican Party took control of Congress in 1994, Republican governors used the opportunity to propose the transformation of the federal Medicaid entitlement into a block grant to the states. The Republican Congress passed such legislation in 1995, and after it was vetoed by President Bill Clinton, proposed it again in 1996. Although the effort ultimately failed, due again to President Clinton's actions, the struggle over the block grant proposal constituted a policy legacy that shaped the characteristics of the State Children's Health Insurance Program when it was enacted in 1997 (Sardell and Johnson 1998). This will be discussed in Chapter 3.

In contrast to the governors, NACHRI supported a strong EPSDT provision because it would ensure the coverage of treatment of children with complex medical conditions. During the last phase of the Medicaid expansion in 1989–1990, when the NGA was no longer supportive of further Medicaid expansions, NACHRI facilitated a Children's Medicaid Coalition of business as well as provider groups. It included the Health Insurance Association of America, the Chamber of Commerce of the United States, Blue Cross and Blue Shield, the American Hospital Association, the American Medical and Dental Associations, as well as CDF, and the AAP. It successfully advocated for a multiyear phase-in of children who were born after October 1983 and lived in families with incomes below the federal poverty level (Pear 1990).

The Nature of the Children's Health Policy Network

Kay Johnson, Dana Hughes, and Sara Rosenbaum (1988) describe the maternal and child health advocacy network as consisting of actors within government, "trade organizations," "religious and voluntary organizations," and "representational groups."[21] The AAP and NACHRI are clearly trade organizations or provider groups, and the March of Dimes is listed in their category of religious and voluntary organizations. Families USA, like CDF, is a "representational group," described as organizations "whose mission is solely their representation of an affected consumer population group" (Johnson, Hughes, and Rosenbaum 1988: 206). Families USA simply seeks to represent a larger group of consumers than does CDF.

The child health policy network that coalesced around the Medicaid eligibility expansions was a "dominant advocacy coalition" in Sabatier's terms because the private research and advocacy organizations, the public commissions, and the supportive members of Congress all shared the view that the health status of low-income children could be improved by providing access to comprehensive health care. They also all agreed that the federal government should have a major role in financing and facilitating the provision of services. It was a coalition in which "everyone viewed Medicaid as the legislative vehicle for effecting policy change that addressed children's access to health care" (Rosenbaum and Sonosky 2001: 99).

The withdrawal of the NGA from support of Medicaid expansion and its advocacy for a Medicaid block grant to the states does represent fragmentation within the coalition. And there was more fragmentation and conflict over the block grant proposal for children's health insurance initiated by CDF and Senator Edward Kennedy. Nevertheless, over time, the private groups and governmental actors supportive of the expansion of children's health insurance continued to share basic principles about the responsibility of the federal government to assure that all children have health insurance coverage and access to care.

This child health policy network was an elite network of think tanks, elected officials and their staffs, foundations, and other private organizations. Although, as Theda Skocpol (1997) argues, these organizations were very different from the membership organizations of parents that initiated earlier social reforms benefiting children and families,[22] many of these national groups had links to state and local groups that included local activists. In addition, child health advocacy in the 1980s was indirectly linked to the social movements of the 1960s. It was a response to the Reagan administration's attempts to reverse the creations of the Great Society and War on Poverty, both responses to the civil rights movement of the 1950s and 1960s. Many of the officials and staffs of these organizations or institutions, such as CDF and Families

USA, had themselves been part of the student, civil rights, and antiwar movements of the 1960s.[23]

As noted above, several of these groups—AAP, NACHRI, the March of Dimes, and Families USA—continued to be the core of the coalition advocating for expansion of health insurance coverage for pregnant women and children. These groups and others testified before the Clinton administration's Task Force on National Health Reform working groups on the specific needs of children within a national health insurance program. But after the Clinton administration's health insurance plan failed to be enacted and Republicans achieved control of Congress in 1994, this coalition was divided about how expanded coverage could and *should* be achieved. When the Children's Defense Fund and Senator Edward Kennedy decided in 1996 that further Medicaid expansions were not politically feasible, they proposed block grants to the states to subsidize private health insurance coverage for low-income children. This was a source of conflict and fragmentation within the dominant advocacy coalition as other advocacy groups and members of Congress viewed this strategy as a threat to the Medicaid program itself. All of these policy events will be discussed in Chapter 3.

There is also evidence that a competing advocacy coalition with core values that were very different from the dominant advocacy coalition also emerged in the area of children's health policy, beginning in the 1980s.

A Competing Advocacy Coalition

This advocacy coalition was composed of interest groups, researchers, and administration officials who believed in conservative social values such as small government and feared that social and health programs funded by the federal government would interfere with the "natural authority" of the patriarchal family. The existence of this competing advocacy coalition is clearly seen in the 1991 Final Report of the National Commission on Children.

The National Commission on Children was a thirty-six-member bipartisan commission initiated by the Reagan administration and charged with making recommendations to the president. The commission examined several areas of policy that affected the lives of US children (education, income support, juvenile justice), but the chapter on health was the only one to include a Minority Chapter in which nine commissioners expressed dissent from the majority report. The views presented in the Minority Chapter were based on very different assumptions than those of the Majority Chapter about the variables affecting the health status of children and the role of government in relation to families. The Majority Chapter shared the core values of the dominant advocacy coalition. The assumptions of the signatories of the Minority Chapter were that the "market," unfettered by government, will produce high-quality health care (National Commission on Children 1991: 167), and that government involvement actually *undermines* child health by "weakening families." An example of the views of the commissioners who signed the Minority Chapter on the relationship between parental "lifestyle" and children's health status is worth quoting directly:

> The importance of the parents' marital status to a baby's health is largely overlooked—race and poverty are commonly blamed for poor infant health and mortality. In fact, a teenage mother who is unmarried and white is more likely to have a low birth weight baby than a teenage mother who is married and black. *Furthermore, babies born to unmarried, college-educated women die in greater proportions than the babies of married, grade-school dropouts.*[24] (National Commission on Children 1991: 162, emphasis added)

There is evidence that policy decisions about children's health related to innovative forms of health care *delivery*—such as home visiting and school-based health clinics—were greatly affected by the existence of this advocacy coalition concerned about social values. For example, while the Subcommittee on Health and the Environment of the House Energy and Commerce Committee held a hearing in 1987 on bills to fund school-based health center demonstration projects, Congressman Waxman decided not to move forward in supporting this model with federal funds. According to a former staff person who worked with Waxman during this period, this was because, "A is for adolescent, A is also for abortion."[25] Liberal members of Congress who were asked to support services that included reproductive health services for adolescents during the 1980s were responding to the "anticipated opposition" of the "conservative values" advocacy coalition.[26] The year before, in 1986, the National Right to Life Trust Foundation had published a book asserting that school-based health clinics would facilitate the performance of abortions in school cafeterias (Glasow 1986).

Limits of time and scope preclude a longer discussion of the ways in which the "culture wars" affected policymaking in the arena of children's health. The issues of contention were health-care delivery models rather than the expansion of health insurance. But it is important to reiterate here that the initial condition under which the bipartisan Medicaid expansion coalition was created in the mid-1980s was an agreement that the issue of insurance coverage for pregnant women and children would be separated from the issue of abortion. Children's health insurance could expand over time because it was isolated from reproductive politics and other culture war and "family" issues that were the concern of the competing child health advocacy coalition.

Framing Investment in Children's Health

One of the major themes of this book is that the policy "frames" used by child health advocates in the 1980s to build a bipartisan coalition supportive of the expansion of Medicaid eligibility continued to be used to argue for the creation of the SCHIP program in 1997 and its reauthorization and expansion in 2007–2009.[27] While the focus was on infant mortality in the 1980s, in the 1990s it shifted to the health of children of all ages and was framed in terms of the "worthiness" of their parents. By 2007, providing health insurance to children was linked to school readiness, and more recently to the prevention and treatment of obesity. However, the frames used to make the argument for public expenditures on children's health insurance are very similar. Next, I will describe these frames.

As discussed above, proposals to expand Medicaid began as policy recommendations for reducing infant mortality in the southern United States. The issue of infant mortality clearly taps into the idea of children as fragile and vulnerable; at-risk newborns are, of course, the most vulnerable of all children. Infant mortality is also a quantifiable problem and one that could be viewed comparatively. The House Select Committee on Children, Youth, and Families reported that the US infant mortality rate was the highest of twenty-one industrialized nations in 1986 and that the black rate was twice that for whites (Staff of House Select Committee on Children, Youth, and Families 1988). A 1988 federal government report said that immunization rates for young children had declined since 1980 and that DPT (diphtheria-pertussis-tetanus) vaccination rates among US children under age one were half that of Western Europe and Israel (OTA 1988).

The magnitude of the problem of infant mortality in the United States was stated very dramatically by the National Commission to

Prevent Infant Mortality in a 1988 report: if the current rate of infant mortality were not reduced, more infants would die between 1988 and 2000 than the total number of battlefield deaths of Americans in the two World Wars, Korea, and Vietnam combined (National Commission to Prevent Infant Mortality 1988: 6).

The first way that infant mortality and childhood illness and disability were framed during the 1980s was as "preventable" and thus as problems that were amenable to solution. Central to US culture is the value of "solving" problems. The second frame was that preventive services were economically wise because they were "cost-effective." Providing preventive and early diagnostic services, it was often said, would save much larger health costs later on. A third frame can be called the "investment in the workforce" or "human capital" frame. This argument is that investment in the health of young children is an investment in a productive workforce that will be competitive in the world economy. These three frames—the "prevention/solvability" frame, the "cost-effectiveness" frame, and the "human capital" frame—are seen in a series of governmental and privately sponsored reports issued in the latter part of the 1980s.

The National Commission to Prevent Infant Mortality frames infant mortality as a solvable problem in comparison to other policy issues: "Unlike other social problems, where cause and effect can blend together to obscure solutions, we know what we can do to halt the tragedy of infant mortality" (National Commission to Prevent Infant Mortality 1988: 10). This theme of "solvability" is also found in the report of the Ford Foundation Project on Social Welfare and the American Future, which was published a year after the National Commission report: "Bringing a healthy baby into the world is something *we know how to do*, but too often in America we fail to do it" (Ford Foundation 1989: 12, emphasis added).

The consensus within the maternal and child health policy network during the second half of the 1980s was that access to prenatal care early in pregnancy would reduce low birth weight and infant mortality, especially in high risk groups, such as young, poor, and African American and Latina women. At the request of the Subcommittee on Health and the Environment of the House Energy and Commerce Committee and the Senate Labor and Human Resources Committee, the Congressional Office of Technology Assessment (OTA) evaluated various strategies to improve children's health. The OTA reviewed fifty-five studies that examined the relationship between infant mortality and prenatal care and found that low birth weight and neonatal mortality could be reduced if women had early and "comprehensive" prenatal care (OTA 1988: 9).

In addition to preventing the tragedy of early death and disability, reductions in infant mortality and the improvement of children's health are also discussed as cost-effective policies. An oft-quoted figure was that for every dollar spent on prenatal care for high-risk women, $3.38 would be saved by not having to provide neonatal care. These data were from a 1985 study by the Institute of Medicine, which was very influential in shaping congressional opinion about the value of expanding Medicaid eligibility for pregnant women and infants (Kosterlitz 1986b). The OTA analyzed the cost impact of Medicaid eligibility for all pregnant women with incomes below the poverty level and concluded that the cost of additional prenatal care would be more than paid for by saving the costs of hospitalization and other health services for low–birth weight infants. The OTA also calculated that childhood immunizations were cost-effective (OTA 1988: 13–14). The National Commission to Prevent Infant Mortality uses OTA data to make this same cost-effectiveness argument (National Commission to Prevent Infant Mortality 1988: 9), an argument also made by the Committee for Economic Development (CED), a corporate group,[28] as well as the Ford Foundation. The Ford Foundation report says,

> We can pay a little now to try and prevent blighted childhoods or we can pay a lot later for the consequences. In other words, money for decent prenatal care, or more than three times as much to deal with low–birth weight infants; several thousand dollars for a good preschool program to open the mind of a ghetto three-year-old, or tens of thousands of dollars to cope with a hardened teenage criminal. (Ford Foundation 1989: 11)

The solvability and cost-effectiveness frames were also used at the state level in the mid-1980s. Governors Michael N. Castle of Delaware and Martha Layne Collins of Kentucky were cochairs of the National Governors Association "campaign" on children's programs. Castle states, "Investing in young children is like compound interest—the benefits, in reduced costs to society, accrue year after year." Governor Collins points out, "It's easier to build successful children than repair men and women. . . . Early childhood programs cost money and sometimes a lot of it. But crime costs more, overcrowded prisons cost more, welfare costs more and undereducation costs more" (Kosterlitz 1986c: 2849).

The other economic argument made was that investment in child health services was investment in the future national workforce. This argument is made explicitly by both the National Commission to Prevent Infant Mortality and the Ford Foundation. The National Commission says that if our infant mortality rate were reduced to that of Japan (the nation with the lowest rate in the world), the additional 20,000 children who survived each year would contribute $10 billion to the economy as workers (National Commission to Prevent Infant Mortality 1988: 10). The Ford Foundation report discusses the need for a highly skilled labor force if the United States is to compete internationally and says, "We ought to invest in human capital with the same entrepreneurial spirit and concern for long-range payoffs that venture capitalists bring to investments in new enterprises" (Ford Foundation 1989: 46).

This set of policy ideas not only was important in influencing policy change in the 1980s but continued to influence policymaking during the next two decades. The same arguments that were made in the effort to expand Medicaid eligibility were used in the policy debates over expanding children's health insurance during the 1990s and the reauthorization of SCHIP in 2007–2009. These will be analyzed in Chapters 3 and 5, respectively. This is an example of what Peterson calls "substantive policy learning," which, along with political interests, informs governmental decisionmaking.

In summary, the policy community concerned with children's health during the latter part of the 1980s focused on infant mortality as a measurable and "solvable" problem and on the expansion of Medicaid eligibility as the policy solution to this problem. Policy entrepreneurs from children's advocacy groups and from inside government (individual governors and governors' organizations and key members of Congress and their staffs) were successful in the effort to make changes in the Medicaid program to expand coverage of pregnant women and children. The policy processes that resulted in these Medicaid expansions were important policy legacies for the creation of SCHIP in 1997. One element of this legacy was the framing that policymakers brought to the discussions of further expansions of children's health coverage (social learning). Another was the success of expanding coverage through a Medicaid structure that insured a legal right to comprehensive services. For some child health advocates, both inside and outside Congress, the Medicaid expansions in the 1980s were a model for future expansions of coverage and services. This aspect of the legacy became a source of conflict with other children's health advocates during the creation of SCHIP.

Notes

1. Earlier political science literature that examined the policy process as it related to child health focused on the implementation of Title V (Maternal and Child Health) programs and the Early Periodic Screening, Diagnosis, and Treatment program within Medicaid (Altenstetter and Bjorkman 1978; Foltz 1982; Goggin 1987).

2. The 1967 enactment of the Early Periodic Screening, Diagnosis, and Treatment program (which requires that states provide comprehensive pediatric services to all Medicaid-eligible children) was a result of the activities of bureaucratic advocates (policy entrepreneurs?) who were motivated by ideological beliefs in "doing good for kids" (Steiner 1976: 223). And the American Academy of Pediatrics appears to have had a relationship with the administrators of the Title V program at least since the late 1940s (Hutchins 1997).

3. Professor Cornel West of Princeton University is also an exemplar of this role in the current period.

4. In 1983, the same year that the House select committee was established, senators Christopher Dodd (D-CT) and Arlen Spector (R-PA) formed the Senate Children's Caucus (Cohen 2001: 76).

5. Interview, Select Committee staff, March 12, 2001.

6. Ibid.

7. Interview, Southern Regional Task Force staff, June 13, 2001.

8. Interview, NGA staff #2, September 14, 2000.

9. For a discussion of the history and policy successes of the National Association of Community Health Centers, see Sardell 1988.

10. The United States Catholic Conference, an organization of US Catholic bishops, other clergy, and lay people was established in 1966 and merged in 2001 with the National Council of Catholic Bishops to form the United States Conference of Catholic Bishops.

11. See Noah (1991) on Waxman's reputation as the member of Congress most responsible for the Medicaid eligibility expansions of the late 1980s.

12. Interview, March of Dimes policy staff, May 17, 1996.

13. See www.aap.org.

14. Interview, AAP staff #1, January 14, 1999.

15. It did not employ any staff until 1974 when a former children's hospital administrator and board member became executive director and ran the organization out of his home for about ten years. In 1984, the organization moved to its current location in Alexandria, Virginia, very close to Washington, DC (interview, NACHRI staff, November 5, 1998). By 1992, it had 125 member hospitals and its board of trustees was organized into six councils, one of which was public policy (NACHRI 1992).

16. Letter to Professor Craig Ramsay from Lawrence A. McAndrews, president and CEO of NACHRI, December 30, 1992. Obtained by the author from Craig Ramsay, Ohio Wesleyan University.

17. Interview, NACHRI staff, November 5, 1998.

18. Ibid.

19. See www.marchofdimes.com.

20. Interview, March of Dimes staff, June 10, 1996.

21. See Johnson (1999) for a discussion of child advocacy at a later point in time, using the same categories.

22. Skocpol and Dickert (2001) describe the economic and social changes within US society that explain why the locally based national civic associations that were advocates for children and families during the nineteenth and first half of the twentieth century have declined. These include the very large increase of women in the workforce, which reduces their time for civic activity, the use of technology and the mass media to recruit individual supporters, and reliance on funding from foundations and wealthy individuals instead of membership dues. These membership-based civic associations have been replaced (since the 1970s) by national professional advocacy organizations that have funders and supporters rather than members and struggle to connect to local constituencies. In their view, the challenges for such groups are to develop linkages with grassroots and community constituencies so that parents and families can be part of children's advocacy.

23. Interview, Families USA staff #1, January 12, 1999; interview, CDF staff #1, February 25, 1999.

24. The reference for this fact was a Chicago newspaper column, which did not reference other sources.

25. Interview, Democratic House staff #2, February 1, 2000, and see Kosterlitz (1986a).

26. See Morone, Kilbreth, and Langwell (2001) for a discussion of morality politics as it affected opposition to school-based health centers at the state level.

27. A caveat is in order here. Although I am analyzing these frames as elements of the policy process, strategies used to gain support from policymakers and the public, this doesn't mean that these frames don't reflect actual data.

28. The CED was a research and educational organization whose trustees included the presidents and board chairs of the largest US corporations. It published a study in 1987 that included a chart of "Cost-Effective Programs for Children," which included WIC, prenatal care, immunizations, as well as education programs. A cost-benefit ratio is given for each program (Committee for Economic Development 1987).

3

Policy Legacies and Political Entrepreneurs: Enacting Children's Health Insurance

On August 5, 1997, President Bill Clinton signed into law the Balanced Budget Act of 1997 and the Revenue Reconciliation Act of 1997, which together contained $48 billion to fund a new federal-state children's health insurance program for ten years. The State Children's Health Insurance Program (SCHIP) authorized the largest amount of federal money for children's health services since the enactment of Medicaid (Pear 1997b) and became a popular program with politicians across the ideological spectrum. Surprisingly, this program was created by a Congress controlled by conservative Republicans committed to limiting government spending and reversing entitlement programs. And while the federal budget deficit had significantly affected congressional decisions on new spending for many years, federal funding for SCHIP was almost five times President Clinton's initial budget request.

The process of policy formulation was remarkably swift, but filled with discord. In January 1997, few believed that children's health insurance legislation was imminent. While the Senate Democratic leadership announced that the issue had very high priority, Democrats were not unified behind a specific policy strategy. Republican leaders would not consider it as an agenda item for the new Congress without consensus on the issue. Yet in a few short months, momentum for such a program developed, and in spite of both inter- and intraparty conflict, a new, large children's health insurance program was enacted.

In this chapter, I explain both *how* this occurred and how the substantive policy outcome—a program in which states would make most decisions about eligibility and benefits—was shaped by a series of policy legacies, the results of previous political and policy events (see Chapter 1). I also describe how the issue of children's health insurance moved to the top of the federal policy agenda in 1997 as a result of another set of policy legacies.

The creation of new programs involves several stages, including the arrival of an issue on the "institutional agenda" (Birkland 2010), as well as legislative formulation and enactment. I first briefly outline the chronology of the enactment of the SCHIP program, and then describe the prior events that created the policy environment within which consideration of children's health insurance occurred. I explain the process by which the issue of children's health insurance advanced toward the "decision agenda" (Birkland 2010), providing part of the answer as to how the SCHIP program was created. The other part of the answer, the variables that made possible the *enactment* of SCHIP, is then discussed. I argue that entrepreneurial activity by a triumvirate of Senator Edward M. Kennedy, Senator Orrin G. Hatch, and the Children's Defense Fund was critical to the creation of a political momentum that moved children's health insurance into the 1997 congressional budget process, while actions by the Clinton administration during the Conference Committee process assured its inclusion in the 1997 Balanced Budget Act (BBA). Finally, I discuss how the characteristics of the first federal legislation explicitly framed as providing health insurance for children were a product of that policy process.

An Overview of the Enactment of SCHIP

By 1997, for a variety of reasons to be discussed here, the issue of "uninsured children" had moved to the decision agenda. In spite of the increase in coverage that resulted from the Medicaid eligibility expansions between 1984 and 1990, 9.6 million or 13 percent of the 71 million children in the United States lacked any health insurance coverage in 1997. Children constituted about a quarter of the uninsured US population. These children were generally in families with working parents; 80 percent of uninsured children had a parent who worked part-time and 60 percent had a parent who worked full-time. While the overall number of uninsured children had grown only slightly since the late 1980s, there had been a 7.1 percent decrease in the percentage of children with private insurance and a 7.6 percent increase in children covered by the Medicaid program. Even though Medicaid coverage for children seemed to be replacing lost private insurance coverage, 3 million children who were eligible for Medicaid were not enrolled in the program.[1]

In his fiscal year 1998 budget proposal sent to Congress on February 6, 1997, President Clinton included several initiatives to reduce the number of uninsured children. First was an effort to reach 1.6 million of the 3 million children eligible for, but not enrolled in, the Medicaid program. A second proposal was to allow states to guarantee Medicaid eligibility to children for one year, reducing movement on and off Medicaid as family income fluctuated. The third proposal was to provide $3.8 billion over five years for grants to states to design programs providing private health insurance for children not eligible for Medicaid. In addition, uninsured children would be included in a four-year demonstration program to provide health insurance for the recently unemployed. The estimated total cost of these initiatives was $11 billion to $12 billion for five years to cover about 5 million of the estimated 10.5 million uninsured kids (Pear 1997a; Nather 1997a).[2] Senate Republicans criticized the administration's proposals as "new entitlements," while congressional Democrats and advocates for children criticized them as too limited (Nather 1997b).[3]

At the beginning of the 105th Congress in 1997, the Senate Democratic minority leader Tom Daschle (ND) announced that children's health insurance was the Democrats' number one health-care issue. Polls suggested that voters supported that priority, but legislators and children's advocates were divided on policy solutions. Three approaches were most often discussed: (1) tax subsidies to individuals to purchase insurance, (2) federal grants to the states, and (3) Medicaid expansions (Nather and Simendinger 1997; BNA 1997a). Republican leaders, who controlled the congressional agenda, would not put children's health insurance on a list of issues for bipartisan action because there was so little consensus on policy solutions (BNA 1997b).

During the first four months of the congressional session, several bills were introduced that aimed to reduce the number of children without health insurance. The sponsors were representatives Pete Stark (D-CA), Frank Pallone Jr. (D-NJ), Marge Roukema (R-NJ), Robert Matsui (D-CA), and Nancy Johnson (R-CT), and senators Daschle, Arlen Spector (R-PA), Phil Gramm (R-TX), Edward M. Kennedy (D-MA), Orrin Hatch (R-UT), John Chafee (R-RI), and John A. Rockefeller (D-WV). The proposed legislation included federal funding for a state voucher program (Specter), federal tax subsidies for families to purchase health insurance for their children (Daschle, Stark), a Medicare-type universal program for all uninsured pregnant women and children financed through a payroll tax (Stark), a federal block grant program to assist states in providing health insurance to children not eligible for Medicaid financed by an increase in the cigarette tax (Kennedy and Hatch, Pallone and Roukema, Johnson and Matsui), an expansion of Medicaid coverage to certain groups of pregnant women and children through an enhanced federal matching grant to the states (Chafee and Rockefeller), and grants to the states through the Title V Maternal and Child Block Grant Program to be used for health care for uninsured children (Gramm) (Johnson et al. 1997).

The State Children's Health Insurance Program, which was established as part of the fiscal year 1998 budget process, was a modified version of the federal block grant program for children's health insurance announced by senators Kennedy and Hatch in March 1997 at the Children's Defense Fund (CDF) annual meeting and introduced into the Senate in April as the Child Health Insurance and Lower Deficit (CHILD) Act. It would provide funding to states for health insurance for children and would be funded with an increase in the cigarette tax.

The enactment of SCHIP followed a pattern in which new domestic programs were created within the context of a two-step reconciliation process established by the 1974 Budget Act in order to limit the size of budget deficits. First, the House and Senate Budget Committees produce a joint budget resolution that sets limits on spending and instructs each committee as to its spending target for the year. The authorizing committees then produce spending and revenue bills, which are included in an omnibus budget reconciliation bill enacted in each House. Then the final Omnibus Budget Reconciliation Act Resolution is negotiated by a House-Senate conference committee. The legislation is debated under rules (particularly in the Senate) that limit the opportunities for changing it outside of committees (Davidson and Oleszek 2002: 387–388). In 1997, the budget resolution included provisions for two reconciliation bills, one for entitlement and program spending (the Balanced Budget Act of 1997) and one for decreases in taxes (the Revenue Reconciliation Act of 1997) (Nather and Teske 1997a).

The authorizing committees that worked on the children's health insurance legislation were the Senate Finance Committee, and initially both the House Commerce[4] and Ways and Means committees.[5] There was a jurisdictional dispute between these committees[6] (Nather 1997d), but Ways and Means lost; the children's health insurance provisions in the House reconciliation legislation were written by the Commerce Committee.

On May 15 a budget agreement was reached between the White House and the Republican congressional leadership that included $16 billion for children's health programs. As the Senate considered this budget deal on May 21, senators Kennedy and Hatch offered an amendment to increase the cigarette tax by $.43 a pack and add $20 billion of the $30 billion raised by the tax increase to the $16 billion already allocated for children's health. The other $10 billion would be for deficit reduction. Republican leaders in the Senate opposed the amendment, as did senators in both parties from tobacco-growing states. The Republican leadership asked their members to vote against it and prevailed upon President Clinton to persuade Democrats to do the same in the interest of preserving the budget agreement. A vote to table the amendment was approved 55–45, with nine Democrats supporting it while seven Republicans defied their leadership to vote with Kennedy and Hatch (Nather and Teske 1997a). However, on June 19, in a surprise move and by a vote of 18–2, the Senate Finance Committee passed a $.20 per pack increase in the tobacco tax advocated by Senator Hatch, a member of the committee. This would add $8 billion to the $16 billion already allocated for children's health (Nather 1997f).[7] The full Senate approved the $.20 tobacco tax increase as part of the tax reconciliation bill, and the $24 billion to be spent for the children's health program (Nather 1997g). The House's allocation remained at $16 billion, but the final conference committee agreement included the $24 billion.

The Clinton administration "pushed" for and won the extra $8 billion in the reconciliation conference committee (Pear 1997b). Within the overall negotiations on the BBA, the children's health insurance program was a high priority for the president and was negotiated at the end of the process, as part of "closing the deal" by the White House and House and Senate leadership. Funding for the program and the substance of the benefits package were both negotiated directly by administration officials and the House and Senate Republican leadership, while White House, Senate, and House staff negotiated issues considered less critical, such as cost-sharing by beneficiaries and state funding formulas.[8] Although there was more intense lobbying on other provisions of the BBA throughout the legislative process, children's health insurance was the "dominant issue" in the conference committee and was "very, very contentious."[9] While the administration "won" on the funding issue, it made compromises on other issues (Nather 1997j). These issues of program design are best understood within the context of the policy legacies that child health advocates, members of Congress, and the White House were all responding to as they interacted to create the SCHIP program.

Children's Health Insurance and the Policy Agenda

Proposals for Expanding Children's Health Insurance Coverage

While participating in efforts to expand Medicaid eligibility, the American Academy of Pediatrics (AAP) also worked to expand coverage of children through private employer-based health insurance plans at the state level.[10] AAP state chapters attempted to persuade state legislators to require that preventive child health care be part of all health insurance plans (Sardell 1991). In 1990, the AAP developed a federal bill that would require employers to extend health insurance to all pregnant women and children up to age 21. Employers who did not comply would pay into a state-administered public plan that would cover those not in employer-sponsored plans. House member Robert Matsui (D-CA) introduced this legislation in 1991, and again in 1993 (American Academy of Pediatrics 1993).

Other kinds of plans to provide universal access to health care for pregnant women and children were also discussed in Congress and the Washington policy community during the early 1990s. Pete Stark, the chairman of the Subcommittee on Health of the Ways and Means Committee introduced a bill to provide universal health insurance for pregnant women and children financed by an increase in the payroll tax equal to the Medicare tax and held hearings on the bill in 1990.[11] Health insurance for children was also on the agenda of two national commissions appointed during the administration of George H. W. Bush. The Advisory Council on Social Security recommended that health insurance be provided to cover all 10 million uninsured children in 1991, but could not reach a consensus on proposals to cover uninsured adults (Pear 1991). The Majority Report of the National Commission on Children recommended that health-care coverage for pregnant women and children be a right of employment (National Commission on Children 1991). A strategy of focusing on health insurance coverage for children as a first step to broader coverage was discussed by health reform advocates *before* the 1992 election, but with the election of Bill Clinton as president, the focus of these advocates moved back to universal coverage (Knox 1994). Most children's advocates, including policy entrepreneurs within Congress, still viewed the Medicaid strategy as the most viable means to expand health coverage for children.

Events during the first half of the 1990s changed the policy environment and power relationships within Congress. When health insurance for children was next on the decision agenda in 1997, the political stream had shifted in a way that precluded the success of federally mandated health insurance proposals such as those of Congressman Stark or the AAP. The failure of the Clinton Health Plan, the 1994 election, and the consequent increased influence of the National Governors Association constitute a series of policy legacies that shaped the characteristics of the new children's health insurance program that was enacted.

Children's Coverage and the Failure of the Clinton Plan

Children's advocates attempted to shape the Clinton administration's Health Security plan, as did other interest groups. Under that plan, most children would be covered by the standard benefit package, comparable to that provided by commercial health insurance companies. But poor children would remain in Medicaid and therefore be guaranteed more comprehensive benefits under the Early Periodic Screening, Diagnosis, and Treatment program. Children's advocates worked with senators Kennedy, Chafee, and Tom Harkin (D-IA) to include in the Health Security plan a long-term care provision for children with special needs who did not qualify for Medicaid (Sardell and Johnson 1998). However, the provisions related to children's coverage became moot when Congress failed to enact health reform. Yet, during the last weeks of the consideration of health reform, children became the focus of the efforts of liberal Democrats to enact proposals that would expand insurance coverage.

The health reform plan introduced by President Clinton in September 1993 threatened the health-care industry with cost controls, was opposed at the local level by activists from small business and the religious right, and was successfully attacked on ideological grounds by conservative intellectuals and Republican leaders at the national level (Skocpol 1997).[12] It was never debated on the floor of the House and did not come to the Senate floor until August 1994. After weeks of unproductive debate, the Senate majority leader, George J. Mitchell (D-ME), proposed a substitute bill that had the support of moderate and liberal Democrats.[13] Another group of senators calling themselves the Mainstream Coalition put forward a bipartisan plan that, unlike the

Mitchell plan, did not include mandated coverage (Rubin and Cloud 1994; Clymer 1999: 544; and see Cloud 1994). While Mitchell was trying unsuccessfully to work out a compromise with the mainstream group, yet another group of senators calling themselves the Children First group proposed a plan to subsidize private health insurance for pregnant women and children in low-income working families who were not eligible for Medicaid.

The Children First group, led by senators Jay Rockefeller, Tom Harkin, and Christopher Dodd (D-CN), proposed a comprehensive benefits package for pregnant women and children that would be financed by an increase in the cigarette tax (Harkin 1994).[14] In addition, a Children First "Dear Colleague" letter was circulated, signed by seventeen senators, stating that any health reform legislation passed by the Senate should include "affordable and accessible health care for children and pregnant women."[15] Although the Children First proposal ultimately fared no better than had the Clinton plan, the focus on children as an incremental strategy, as well as the nature of the proposal itself, foreshadowed the successful enactment of SCHIP in 1997.[16]

In October 1994, Robert Pear, the *New York Times* health policy reporter, described a general belief in the need for incrementalism on health reform. Pear noted that "one area of obvious political appeal is legislation to assure health care for children" (Pear 1994: A3). While the issue of health insurance coverage for children had been discussed within the children's (and broader) health policy community before the formulation of the Clinton plan in 1993, it was the failure of the Clinton plan that created an "incrementalist" stance among congressional liberals and health activists. As a result of years of "softening-up" activity (Kingdon 1995: 127–130) on children's health issues by the child health policy community, covering uninsured children was an obvious answer when other political actors asked, "What is the next incremental step we can take toward increased health care access?" This follows the pattern of events in 1951, when a group of President Harry Truman's advisers developed an incremental strategy of seeking limited hospital coverage for Social Security beneficiaries when it became clear that Congress was not going to pass Truman's national health insurance plan (Marmor 2000).

Problem Definition at the State and Federal Levels

By the winter of 1996–1997, many state and federal policymakers were convinced that a lack of health insurance for children was a growing problem. A higher proportion of children than adults had lost private health coverage, and structural changes in the economy indicated that a loss of employment-related health insurance would continue. Changes in the welfare system might increase the number of children not covered at all, as families lost Medicaid along with their welfare coverage but were not able to find employment that provided health insurance to replace it (Burns 1997). As noted earlier, it was only the expansion of Medicaid coverage for pregnant women and children during the latter part of the 1980s that kept the number of uninsured children from growing even more rapidly. Of the estimated 10.5 million uninsured children in 1995, 80 percent lived in families with incomes at or below 250 percent of the federal poverty level (FPL) (GAO 1996).

A large number of studies and reports also discussed the links between insurance coverage and health services utilization among children, the low cost of care for children as compared to adults, and the long-term cost-effectiveness of preventive care for children (see Holahan 1997). In addition to studies documenting the benefits of health insurance coverage for children, there were also activities within the states that federal policymakers could point to as policy models.

By 1997, some effort to increase health insurance coverage for children had been made in all but six states. Some state governments had attempted to directly subsidize the purchase of health insurance by small businesses or to provide tax credits or vouchers to uninsured families, but the larger efforts to cover uninsured children involved expansions of Medicaid eligibility beyond federally mandated levels, activities to increase the enrollment of Medicaid eligible children, and the establishment of separate state-funded children's health insurance programs. Thirty-seven states had used the state Medicaid option to expand coverage for pregnant women and children above the federally required income level, while eight states had established state-funded programs for children with family incomes above the Medicaid eligibility level (Johnson and McDonough 1998).

A key political link between these state experiences and entrepreneurial efforts at the federal level on behalf of children's health insurance was the introduction of two health insurance proposals by Senator John Kerry (D-MA) in 1996. In June, Kerry proposed to subsidize health insurance coverage for children in "working families" with incomes between 185 percent and 300 percent of the FPL and to provide a "comprehensive benefits package" that would include pregnancy-related services through subsidies and/or vouchers on an income-based sliding scale.[17] Three months later, at the end of the 104th Congress, Senator

Kerry along with Senator Edward Kennedy introduced into the Senate the "Family Values Child Health Insurance Act." This was basically the same proposal with the more explicit directive that states administering the program would contract with private insurance companies to provide coverage for children and pregnant women. Families with incomes below 185 percent of the FPL would be fully subsidized, while those with incomes between 185 percent and 300 percent of the FPL would receive subsidies on a sliding-scale basis. The plan was to be financed by "closing corporate loopholes" and increasing the tobacco tax.

The impetus for the introduction of this bill was Senator Kerry's close reelection battle with Governor William Weld in Massachusetts. Governor Weld had vetoed a state child health insurance bill based on his opposition to the cigarette tax that was to finance it. (His veto was subsequently overridden by the Massachusetts legislature in July of 1996 [BNA 1996: 1225].) Senator Kerry's sponsorship of a children's health insurance bill at the federal level was, according to one former legislative aide, "an opportunity for Senator Kerry to say to Governor Weld 'are you for the big tobacco companies or are you for kids?'"[18] This was also the major theme used to mobilize support for similar legislation introduced by senators Kennedy and Hatch during the 105th Congress.

There were other direct links between policy entrepreneurs acting on the children's health insurance issue in Massachusetts with policy entrepreneurs at the federal level. At the beginning of their efforts to enact a major children's health insurance program in Massachusetts, state legislator John McDonough, the chief architect of the initiative, and his allies asked the Kerry Senate campaign to discuss the issue in order to focus attention on it in the state. After achieving success in creating a children's health insurance program financed in part by a tobacco tax, these policy entrepreneurs at the state level urged Senator Kennedy to use this model at the federal level (McDonough 2000).

Thus, the policy legacy of agenda-building for children's health (as part of a focus on children's needs in general) during the 1980s, combined with the failure of the attempt to create universal health insurance in 1994, resulted in *a focus on children* by members of Congress concerned about expanding coverage. Yet the *substance* of these proposals was shaped by a separate series of policy events. These were the 1994 congressional election and the subsequent near-successful attempt by Republican governors to radically change the nature of the Medicaid program.

Policy Formulation:
The Legacy of the Medicaid Block Grant Battle

Proposals to replace the federal entitlement to Medicaid with a block grant to the states came close to being enacted in 1995–1996. Although Medicaid survived as an entitlement program, the legacy of this block grant debate shaped the policy environment in which children's health insurance legislation was proposed, debated, and enacted in 1997. The concerns of key actors in the 1995–1996 Medicaid block grant debate were central to the policy process of enacting the children's health insurance legislation, and their influence is visible in its policy outcomes.

In the election of 1994, the Republicans won both houses of Congress for the first time since the 83rd Congress (1953–1955). Thirty-four Democratic members of the House were defeated, and seventy-three new Republican members took office in January 1995. The programmatic center of the Republican campaign, led by Congressman Newt Gingrich (R-GA), was the reduction of federal spending for social programs and balancing the federal budget. It was dramatized by the signing of the Contract with America on the Capitol steps of the House in September 1994 (Davidson and Oleszek 2002).

As discussed in Chapter 2, the National Governors Association had been part of the coalition that successfully advocated for the expansion of Medicaid eligibility for pregnant women and children during the 1980s. But by the end of the decade, the governors, particularly Republican governors, opposed the further expansion of Medicaid eligibility and also called for the repeal of the Early Periodic Screening, Diagnosis, and Treatment Program (EPSDT) program. During the 104th Congress (1995–1997), Republican governors (who also became a majority of state executives) enjoyed considerable access to the Republican congressional leadership. At the governors' request, legislation was introduced in 1995 and 1996 that would replace the existing Medicaid entitlement program with a block grant to the states. Most decisions about Medicaid eligibility and benefits would be made at the state level.

Children's advocates generally opposed the Medicaid block grant proposal and worked against it from within a broad anti–block grant coalition, which included senior citizens groups, religious groups, advocates for persons with disabilities, professional associations, and provider groups, many of whom would be affected by a restructuring of Medicaid.

The Republican-controlled Congress passed the legislation, but it was vetoed by President Clinton in December 1995. A second effort by the governors to "reform Medicaid" failed in 1996 when President Clinton asked the Republican congressional leadership to choose between restructuring Medicaid or welfare. They opted to drop the Medicaid issue in favor of the more salient issue of "welfare reform" (Sardell and Johnson 1998).

The policy legacy of the Medicaid block grant battle can be seen in the fact that only two of the bills introduced to deal with the problem of uninsured children during the winter of 1997 called for an expansion of a federal entitlement to health insurance coverage. All of the others used either a tax credit, a voucher plan, or a block grant to the states as the mechanism for establishing a state-administered program to enroll uninsured children in private health insurance plans. With the exception of Congressman Stark's proposal for a Medicare program for pregnant women and children, all of the proposals assumed the devolution of power to the states. Only Chafee and Rockefeller sought to expand the Medicaid program, but this was to be done by offering an option linked to financial rewards to the states rather than as a federal requirement. Even Senator Kennedy, a longtime, energetic advocate of federally sponsored universal health coverage, was in 1997 proposing a plan for block grants to the states.

The Hatch-Kennedy bill was controversial within the child health policy community, and this was also a legacy of the Medicaid block grant battle. Staff of advocacy groups and some members of Congress and their staffs believed that the enactment of a block grant would begin a process of weakening and eventually dismantling Medicaid as a vehicle for providing federal health insurance to low-income children.[19] They supported bills sponsored by senators Chafee and Rockefeller that further expanded Medicaid. The dominant child health advocacy coalition was thus divided over whether Medicaid expansion should continue to be the vehicle for expanding coverage of uninsured children. The two provider associations that advocated for expansion of children's health coverage—the American Academy of Pediatrics and the National Association of Children's Hospitals—supported the block grant proposal, but groups concerned about health-care access for all low-income populations, such as the Center on Budget and Policy Priorities and Families USA, did not. Officials and staff of these organizations were afraid that the block grant strategy posed a threat to the very structure of health-care entitlements (Rosenbaum and Sonosky 2001).

Congressional staff and staff of advocacy groups expressed frustration that although they had worked very hard in 1995 and 1996 to defeat the NGA Medicaid block grant proposal, the Hatch-Kennedy bill meant that now "the governors had come back." There was a "line in the sand" about preserving the Medicaid entitlement that Kennedy and Hatch were crossing.[20] Some policy actors suggested that the existence of the Hatch-Kennedy bill made it politically impossible to get a Medicaid expansion: "Kennedy initiated it, compromised and doomed it to a block grant all at the same time."

In spite of these tensions within the policy community, Medicaid advocates and supporters of the block grant approach decided that the Chafee-Rockefeller and Kennedy-Hatch proposals could complement each other. Advocates for each approach agreed to support both approaches throughout the congressional process.[21] Both Hatch and Kennedy were cosponsors of the Chafee-Rockefeller bill.

The influence that the NGA had on health-care issues during the 104th Congress continued during the 105th, a Congress in which the Republicans again controlled the majority of seats. The primary objective of the NGA throughout the process of consideration of children's health insurance was to insure state flexibility over critical decisions such as benefits eligibility and provider networks (see Nather 1997h), a goal supported by Republicans on the House Energy and Commerce Committee.[22] At a hearing held by the Senate Finance Committee entitled *Governors' Perspective on Medicaid,* the only two witnesses, Governor Bob Miller of Nevada, the chair of the NGA, and Governor Michael O. Leavitt of Utah, a member of the NGA's Medicaid Task Force, discussed the NGA's positions on Medicaid.[23]

The organization was opposed to President Clinton's proposal for a per capita Medicaid cap as a way to reduce the growth of Medicaid spending and to any mandatory Medicaid eligibility expansion. The two governors also proposed eliminating the federal waiver needed to enroll Medicaid recipients in managed care and repeal of both the Boren amendment, which required states to reimburse nursing homes and hospitals at "reasonable and adequate rates" under the Medicaid program, and cost-based reimbursement of federally qualified community health centers.[24] They also called for an examination of the difference in cost between an actuarially based package of benefits and those offered under EPSDT.[25] As I discuss below, the BBA of 1997 gave the governors most of what they wanted in relationship to the Medicaid program.

The Senate Process

The three children's health plans initially competing in the Senate Finance Committee were Republican senator Phil Gramm's proposal to expand the Title V Maternal and Child Health (MCH) program, the Kennedy-Hatch CHILD bill, and the bipartisan Chafee-Rockefeller proposal to expand eligibility for Medicaid coverage to children in families with incomes up to 150 percent of the FPL (Nather 1997f; Nather and Teske 1997b). Thus, key Republicans on the Finance Committee were divided on the issue of children's health insurance. Chafee was advocating for the Medicaid expansion, Hatch for the CHILD bill. Senator Don Nickles of Oklahoma, who was part of the Senate Republican leadership, initially opposed any new program for children's health insurance, believing that the number of uninsured children was overstated. When it was clear that there would be a bill, Senator Nickles acted to ensure state accountability by requiring that additional funding for a children's health insurance program be used to cover new children, not children who were already eligible for Medicaid.[26] This concern was the basis for the provision in the SCHIP legislation that states with separate children's insurance programs (see below) are not allowed to enroll Medicaid-eligible children in that program. Republican members of the Finance Committee were also concerned about "crowd-out" (the substitution of public coverage for private insurance), and there was "great discomfort" when proposals to cover children in higher-income families were discussed.[27]

When the Medicaid expansion proposal was put before the Finance Committee on June 17, the committee (in a very close vote of 9 to 11) rejected a modified plan sponsored by Senator Chafee to use $12 billion of the $16 billion allocated for children's health in the budget agreement to provide Medicaid coverage to all children living in households with incomes up to 133 percent of the FPL (Nather 1997f). This proposal would have gone beyond the Medicaid phase-in for fourteen- to eighteen-year-olds living in households with incomes at or below 100 percent of the FPL that was to be completed by 2002. Chafee, Rockefeller, and their staffs believed that the Chafee amendment would pass because they had been promised the support of nine Democrats and four Republicans on the Committee—Hatch, James Jeffords, Chafee, and Alfonse D'Amato.

During interviews more than a year later, former staff members still discussed this reversal in the committee with strongly negative feelings—"the most dirty politics I've ever seen . . . the worst in nine years on the Hill," according to one interviewee. Congressional committee staff also stated that some of the committee members who had originally supported the Chafee proposal changed their votes when Republican leaders gave them—Democrats as well as Republicans—"gifts from the BBA legislation." Governors, particularly Republican governors, also "put a lot of pressure" on the senators from their states. A longtime Republican House staff member recalled that this was a "key vote." "If that vote had gone the other way, it would have been an open question whether this would have been a block grant or a Medicaid expansion."[28]

The chair of the Senate Finance Committee, William Roth (R-DE), responded to these divisions within the committee by crafting a compromise that allowed states to either expand Medicaid or establish a separate program to cover uninsured children.[29] This provision was retained in the final legislation. The Kennedy-Hatch bill required that the EPSDT program be included in all state health plans. This requirement was dropped during Senate Finance Committee deliberations. Instead, the final Senate bill required that the benefit packages provided by the states offer the same benefits as those offered in Blue Cross and Blue Shield plans, with the addition of hearing and vision services. The inclusion of these services was authored by Senator Chafee and proposed on the Senate floor as part of a substitute children's health plan by Senator Roth (Nather and Teske 1997c).

The Process in the House

The Ways and Means Committee. Although the House bill came out of the Commerce Committee, the only House hearing on children's health insurance was held on April 8 by the Health Subcommittee of the Ways and Means Committee, which initially competed with the Energy and Commerce Committee for jurisdiction.[30] The content of this hearing, held after several children's health insurance bills had been introduced into the 105th Congress, reflected concern about the relationship between private and public insurance.

The purpose of the hearing was to have policy experts from both government (the Congressional Budget Office, the Congressional Research Service, the Government Accounting Office) and private think tanks (the Urban Institute, the Institute for Health Policy Solutions, and the National Bureau of Economic Research) summarize their research findings on the number and characteristics of uninsured children, the reasons why they were uninsured, the relationship between health insurance coverage and access to health care, and the consequences of various policy options to increase the number of insured children. Two of the central issues in the presentations and discussions with subcommittee members were the 3 million uninsured children who were eligible for Medicaid but not enrolled, and the possibility of "crowd-out."[31] The experts differed as to the income level at which crowd-out occurs, support for policies to reduce crowd-out (such as waiting periods for public coverage and copayments), and the level of crowd-out they believed was acceptable in order to pursue broader policy goals such as improving children's health. There was agreement that the crowd-out effect was most likely to occur as family income rises, especially above 200 percent of the FPL.

Another concern voiced by Health Subcommittee Chair Bill Thomas was that the benefits available in a public insurance program might be "richer" than the benefits offered by private insurance plans. This was also a problem identified by Representative Nancy L. Johnson, a Republican subcommittee member who took a leadership role on this issue in the House. As mentioned earlier, representatives Johnson and Robert Matsui, a Democratic colleague on the Ways and Means Committee, had introduced a bill into the House that was almost identical to the Kennedy-Hatch bill with the exception of the benefits package. The Johnson-Matsui bill did not include EPSDT as part of its benefit structure, but rather required states to provide benefit packages that were comparable to the Blue Cross and Blue Shield Federal Employees Health Benefits plan. Congresswoman Johnson believed that states should have "flexibility" in making benefit decisions and did not want to "prescribe" public benefits for children that were more generous than those offered by employers to other working parents.[32]

Underlying these concerns was the assumption that while government might subsidize health insurance coverage for those outside the private, employment-based system, the public sector should never "compete" with the private sector but rather help to maintain it. This is the conceptual/ideological boundary between public and private programs that I discussed in Chapter 1. This "boundary" was central in policy conflict over SCHIP reauthorization a decade later in 2007.

The Commerce Committee. The Commerce Committee bill was written by the Republican majority staff working with NGA staff.[33] The Democratic members of the Commerce Committee proposed a Medicaid expansion like the Chafee-Rockefeller proposal in the Senate, but it was rejected along party lines. The Democrats then voted for the Republican chair's proposal or "mark" because they did not want to be seen as voting against children's health legislation.[34] The House bill reflected the NGA's position on benefits. It required that states cover only four basic categories of service: (1) inpatient and outpatient hospital services, (2) physician's services, (3) laboratory and x-ray services, (4) well-baby and well-child care, including immunizations (Nather 1997h).

The Conference Committee

As I discussed in the overview of the SCHIP legislative process, the Clinton administration played a major role in the contentious 1997 BBA conference committee negotiations on the children's health insurance program. The administration succeeded in having the higher funding level in the Senate bill included in the final legislation but did not prevail on the benefits issue. The politics of the benefit provisions, as of the conference committee generally, was that the White House, congressional Democrats, and moderate Republicans supported the Senate version of the child health bill and the Republican leadership and the NGA supported the House version. Senator Roth, the chairman of the Senate Finance Committee, argued for the Senate benefit provisions against the Republican leadership. As earlier in the process, there was conflict among Senate Republicans.

A bipartisan group of governors met privately with members of the conference committee on July 15 and argued that the House version of the bill would allow states to cover more children because they would save money on benefits. Governor Bob Miller, Democrat of Nevada, made the same argument to the Clinton administration. Children's advocates, Democrats, and moderate Republicans such as Senator Chafee argued, in contrast, that the Senate bill contained the minimum necessary benefit package to assure that children would receive adequate health services. At one point the Senate Republican leadership proposed that the Senate benefit provision be replaced with seven possible options from which states could choose. Significantly, in terms of the NGA's opposition to EPSDT and its effort to convert Medicaid to a block grant in 1995 and 1996, one of these options was "all Medicaid benefits except EPSDT" (Nather 1997i).

In the compromise agreement reached during the negotiations, the Clinton administration agreed to greater state flexibility in the benefit structure than had been contained in the Senate bill. The legislation that was enacted gave the states a choice of three "benchmark" benefit plans: the Blue Cross and Blue Shield preferred provider organization (PPO) plan used by federal employees, a state employee health plan, or the health maintenance organization (HMO) in the state with the largest private sector enrollment. It then allowed the states to create their own plan as long as it had the same actuarial value as one of these plans or the approval of the Department of Health and Human Services (DHHS). It did require that any state plan provide the specific four service categories included in the House bill; in addition, if an actuarial equivalent plan was chosen, hearing, vision, prescription drug, and mental health benefits had to be provided at 75 percent of the value of the plan used to determine equivalent value (Nather 1997j). This benefit provision clearly represented the stated interests of the NGA for state autonomy.

The success of the governors in achieving their policy objectives in the 1997 BBA went beyond the structure of the children's health insurance program. At the same time that SCHIP was enacted, many changes were made in the Medicaid program that the NGA had sought for years, including state ability to mandate the enrollment of Medicaid beneficiaries in managed care without federal waivers, the repeal of the Boren amendment, and the phasing out of cost-based reimbursement of federally qualified community health centers and rural health clinics (Nather 1997k). In a sense, the children's health insurance and Medicaid portions of the spending and tax legislation enacted in 1997 can be seen as a victory for the NGA in the battle in which they were engaged during the debate about the Medicaid block grant in 1995 and 1996.

The Dynamic of Entrepreneurial Activity

By April of 1997, when Kennedy and Hatch introduced their children's health insurance bill and a related revenue bill there was great interest in the issue of expanding children's health coverage, but a lack of agreement on how it should be done (Hosansky 1997). The dynamic that moved children's health insurance to enactment as part of the Balanced Budget Act of 1997 was the successful entrepreneurial strategy of Senator Edward Kennedy and the Children's Defense Fund. That strategy had three parts: (1) the substance of the proposal itself, (2) bipartisan and cross-ideological sponsorship, and (3) the framing of the bill.

The Substance of the Proposal

As I have discussed, the Hatch-Kennedy bill, like the Kerry-Kennedy bill that preceded it, was a federal grant to the states for the purchase of children's health insurance financed by an increase in the cigarette tax. Like almost all of the health insurance proposals introduced into the 105th Congress, it was not an individual entitlement to health insurance coverage as was Medicaid. Democratic congressional leaders were supporting an income tax credit for the purchase of health insurance for children, but Senator Kennedy and his staff believed that the children's health insurance programs already operating in several states would be a less expensive and more efficient way of reaching low-income families with uninsured children.[35] In fact, Kennedy and his staff acted as both "policy" and "politics" entrepreneurs within their own party on children's health insurance (Peterson 1997: 1090). They urged Democratic leaders and the Clinton administration to make the issue a priority, and they argued within the Democratic Party for a state block grant approach rather than for the income tax credit proposals that were being developed by the Democratic leadership.[36]

The Children's Defense Fund was the leader of the nongovernmental actors advocating for the Medicaid expansions during the 1980s, and its priority in health care in the mid-1990s was still a large expansion in health insurance coverage for children. In 1996, national focus group research commissioned by a consultant hired by CDF to examine how children's health issues could fit within the election year political agenda found public support for children's health insurance but suggested that a large, new Medicaid expansion was not possible in the existing political environment.[37] However, the CDF leadership believed that the 105th Congress presented an opportunity to push children's health issues "as the next phase of incremental health reform."[38] CDF, like Kennedy, was opposed to the tax credit idea.[39]

In Peterson's terms, the promotion of the block grant proposal drew on substantive learning because it was based on successful child health insurance programs in several states. At the same time, Senator Kennedy and the CDF leadership believed the block grant proposal would fit within the policy environment that was created when the Republican Party, led by its conservative wing, won control of the Congress in 1994. They were thus basing their entrepreneurial efforts on judgments about what was politically viable (situational learning).

A Strategy of Bipartisanship

The second part of the strategy that Senator Kennedy used to advance the children's health insurance legislation was bipartisan sponsorship and support in Congress. Kennedy had been the major congressional activist on universal health insurance during his almost thirty-five years in the Senate (see Clymer 1999). Right after the 1994 election, Kennedy and his staff began thinking about covering children as an incremental step toward providing health insurance for the uninsured. They contacted several possible Republican cosponsors but found them uniformly uninterested in new spending within a new Congress committed to ending the deficit.[40] Instead, Senator Kennedy worked with Senator Nancy Kassebaum (R-KS) to sponsor the Health Insurance Portability and Accountability Act of 1996, which established federal standards for health insurance coverage for both insurance companies and self-insured businesses (Markus 1996). This bipartisan and incremental legislation, initiated by Senator Kennedy, was viewed by the senator and his staff as a successful model for operating within the Republican-controlled Congress after the failure of the Clinton health-reform effort.[41] The passage of this legislation also moved congressional Democrats, advocacy groups, and the Clinton administration to consider children's health insurance as the next incremental step (Nather 1996).

Kennedy did cosponsor a children's insurance bill with Senator Kerry at the end of the 104th Congress in 1996, but this was not a politically viable legislative strategy because the bill's sponsors were two liberal Democratic senators from the same state. In planning for the next Congress, Kennedy again began looking for a Republican cosponsor with interest in child health and this time got a positive response from Senator Hatch, a conservative with whom he had often worked on health issues. Kennedy was here acting as an entrepreneur in recruiting others as "investors" (Oliver and Paul-Shaheen 1997). The initial staff contacts were in December of 1996; by January 1997, serious negotiations had begun. "Intense," full-time staff negotiations were held for two months. On March 13, Kennedy and Hatch announced the outlines of their bill at CDF's annual meeting (Pear 1997b) and continued to work out the details. On April 8, 1997, they introduced the Child Health Insurance and Lower Deficit (CHILD) Act into the Senate.[42] Both Kennedy and Hatch made concessions in negotiating the form of their plan.

The major issues during the negotiations were whether children's health insurance would be an entitlement and what the benefits package would contain.[43] Kennedy agreed not to insist on an entitlement to children's health insurance, to reduce the overall amount of money from that in the Kerry-Kennedy bill, and to dedicate one-third of the money raised by the cigarette tax to deficit reduction. Senator Hatch believed that having a substantial portion of the money targeted to deficit reduction would make it harder for Republicans to oppose it.[44] Hatch agreed to a large health insurance program for children financed with a cigarette tax. As a conservative Republican, Hatch was generally opposed to raising taxes. In this case, however, he viewed taxes on cigarettes as justified because of the damaging health effects of smoking (Pear 1997b). After some "very spirited negotiation," Hatch agreed that the benefit package in the bill would be the same as the EPSDT Medicaid benefits.[45]

While Kennedy was the initial congressional politics and policy entrepreneur in moving the legislation that became SCHIP, Hatch's role was very important in its enactment. Hatch was a conservative Republican who had seniority, was a respected legislator, and was a member of the Senate Finance Committee, which had jurisdiction over the legislation. (Kennedy was not a member of the Finance Committee.) Hatch provided bipartisan, "trans-ideological" support for the proposal, and this made it politically viable.[46] A House Republican staff member remarked, "A guy that deserves a lot of credit is Hatch. Hatch went with Kennedy early. . . . He probably deserves more credit for this than anyone else."[47]

Senator Hatch became very knowledgeable about the details of the CHILD legislation and energetically advocated for the legislation within the Republican caucus, arguing that it was in the interest of the Republican Party to support health insurance for children. He recruited several key Republican senators as cosponsors: Ted Stevens of Alaska, chair of the Senate Appropriations Committee; James Jeffords of Vermont, chair of the Labor Committee and a member of the Finance Committee; Olympia Snowe and Susan Collins of Maine; Bob Smith of Oregon; Robert Bennett of Utah; and Ben Nighthorse Campbell of Colorado.[48]

The Republican Party leadership opposed Hatch's position and the Hatch-Kennedy bill. Trent Lott, the Senate majority leader, called it "another big government program takeover that costs billions of dollars when there are other solutions that would get the job done better, helping parents to help their children, taking advantage of existing laws" (BNA 1997c: 579). The Senate leadership asked Republican senators not to cosponsor the bill, and Republican leaders and conservative interest groups attacked Hatch for his legislative partnership with Kennedy.

The Republican Party in Utah voted to censure him.[49] Some of the other Republican senators that Hatch recruited to support the bill were attacked in radio ads sponsored by an organization called Citizens for a Sound Economy, which received donations from large cigarette companies (*Oregonian* 1997; and see Clymer 1999: 587–588).

In May 1997, after the Kennedy-Hatch amendment to increase the cigarette tax by $.43 was defeated on the Senate floor, Senator Hatch argued forcefully within the Senate Finance Committee for a smaller cigarette tax increase of $.20 and prevailed by a vote of 18–2. Several Republican members who had previously been in opposition voted for the increase.[50] As noted earlier, this added another $8 billion to the $16 billion already allocated for children's health insurance and was approved by the full Senate as part of the tax reconciliation bill. Senators Kennedy and Hatch both approached Republican Congresswoman Nancy Johnson to recruit her on behalf of their bill. Johnson responded enthusiastically, cosponsoring a similar bill in the House and pushing the legislation in both letters and conversations with senior Republicans on the Commerce Committee and in the Republican caucus.[51] In this way, Johnson acted as a political entrepreneur for the legislation within the House.

Framing SCHIP:
"Hard-Working Families" vs. "Big Tobacco"

The third part of the Kennedy-Hatch-CDF entrepreneurial strategy was framing the Hatch-Kennedy children's health insurance legislation in a way that would attract support, or "marketing" it (Oliver and Paul-Shaheen 1997). As discussed previously, Medicaid expansion was framed in terms of the cost-effectiveness of the prevention of infant mortality and childhood disease as well as the innocence and vulnerability of children. In response to a long period of education by the child health policy community, both Republican and Democratic members of Congress accepted the idea that children's health services were uniquely cost-effective. The idea that access to health services for children was a means of preventing future costly health conditions, as well as an investment in the US labor force, was "social learning" that continued to influence policy actors in the deliberations over proposed child health insurance legislation in 1997, again across ideological lines.

Bill Thomas, the Republican chairman of the Health Subcommittee of the Ways and Means Committee, referred during the committee's hearing on children's health insurance to "the payoff in terms of dealing with health care early over the life of the child."[52] One of the witnesses at the hearing, Linda Bilheimer of the Congressional Budget Office, reiterated characteristics of children's health services that were part of the basic "policy knowledge" underlying efforts to expand insurance coverage: that preventive care is optimal for children's health, that children without health insurance don't have access to preventive care, and that children are "a relatively inexpensive group of the population to insure."[53] Congresswoman Nancy Johnson argued in support of her version of the Hatch-Kennedy legislation within the Republican caucus in 1997 by stressing the preventive and therefore cost-effective nature of children's health care.[54] Building upon this general support for children's health care, the advocates of both the Kerry-Kennedy bill and the Hatch-Kennedy CHILD bill also framed their proposals as fitting within mainstream US values: rewards for hard work, parental responsibility, limited government, and support of the private sector. In addition, they framed them as a struggle between innocent, vulnerable children and the cigarette companies.

In his statement accompanying the introduction of the Kerry-Kennedy bill, Senator Kennedy stated that the program "is a reflection of true family values" and "does not substitute for family responsibility, but fosters it, by assuring that every family has the help it needs to purchase affordable health insurance for its children." In addition, he emphasized, "Our plan will establish no massive new Federal bureaucracy."[55] Senator Hatch used almost the same words ("it will not create massive, new bureaucracies") in his speech introducing the bill at the March CDF annual meeting.[56] Children's health insurance was framed as a benefit for "working families" to clearly distinguish it from a "welfare benefit."

A CDF official is quoted by a journalist as saying, "Once the public learns that millions of parents who get up every morning and go to work to pay their bills still can't provide health care for their children, they'll hold Congress to a very high standard in solving this problem" (Serafini 1997: 571). In his remarks to CDF, Hatch said,

> Our legislation will help working families across the United States. After all, these are the people who face the world everyday, meeting the challenges of life, working hard, pursuing a better life, and playing by the rules. The Hatch/Kennedy bill will provide a cushion for these families—a cushion that could make a difference between a healthy child or a sick child. As a nation—indeed as a society—we have a moral responsibility to provide that needed layer of support. (Remarks by Senator Hatch, March 13, 1997)

Thus, the problem was defined as not merely the existence of a large number of uninsured children in the United States, but the existence of a large number of uninsured children whose parents were hard working and thus, by implication in the era of welfare "reform," deserving of assistance.

CDF officials and staff wanted to frame the issue of health insurance for children in a way that bypassed negative feelings about entitlements and built on positive attitudes toward working parents. This formulation was based in part on findings from their 1996 focus group research that found negative feelings about "entitlement programs," and also on support for the idea that if working families did not get health insurance through their employers, government should subsidize their health insurance.[57]

The Hatch-Kennedy child health bill was also framed as part of a moral crusade against cigarette companies and smoking by young people. The coalition organized by CDF to support the legislation in the Senate and then to support the Senate position in the conference committee went outside the traditional children's health coalition of children's advocacy groups and health-care providers. Instead, its core groups were antismoking groups such as the American Cancer Society, the American Lung Association, and Tobacco Free Kids. The two primary lobbying strategies used by this coalition were getting media attention for the legislation and mobilizing grassroots antismoking and children's activists at the state and local levels to come to Washington to meet with their legislators. Senate Republicans not supportive of the proposal were initially targeted.[58] The CHILD proposal, and later the Senate bill, was framed as representing a powerful good—the health of children—and at the same time, opposition to a powerful evil—smoking by children and adolescents. "Children's health was popular, reducing smoking was popular, but putting good vs. evil together . . . was about as good as it gets in politics."[59] Many of the ads sponsored by the coalition featured a picture of a young boy and the image of "Joe Camel" with the words underneath, "Joey vs. Joe Camel." A *New York Times* editorial commented, "The Kennedy-Hatch tax would improve health by covering children while discouraging smoking. This is an attractive combination" (*New York Times* 1997). Commenting on the initial defeat of the Hatch-Kennedy amendment to the budget resolution that would raise the cigarette tax to finance children's health insurance, *USA Today* said, "There's just no way to weigh tobacco against medical care for kids in favor of the former. Just. No. Way" (*USA Today* 1997). The *Washington Post* referred to "the young people who the cigarette companies try so hard to hook" and to the fact that the outcome of the implementation of the Kennedy-Hatch proposal would be the expansion of health insurance coverage and a decrease in teen smoking as "a twofer" (*Washington Post* 1997).

Staff for the Republican leadership noted that the framing of health insurance for children in these terms made it very difficult to oppose this legislation, or to appear to be supporting "Joe Camel" over Joey.[60] Part of the explanation for the unusually swift enactment of SCHIP, in spite of conflict over substantive policy questions, was this framing strategy—linking antitobacco sentiment with positive feelings about children, particularly vulnerable children lured into disease-producing behavior by evil tobacco companies. This was the politics of morality writ large, a morality with simple icons of good and evil.

It is important to note another policy legacy related to the framing of SCHIP that was discussed by several congressional staff members during my interviews with them: Congressman Henry Waxman's entrepreneurship on the issue of tobacco during the early 1990s. Beginning with the Senate Children First group in 1994, all of the proposals for children's health insurance (outside of the Medicaid program) were to be financed with increases in the cigarette tax. The hearings held by Congressman Waxman on the activities of the cigarette companies helped to create a negative image of the industry. Senators Hatch and Kennedy and CDF used the negative image of this tobacco policy monopoly to build support for children's health insurance.

In the next phase of policymaking for children's health insurance, rhetoric about US values was again part of the process, but this time it was President George W. Bush and his supporters who argued that expanding publicly supported health insurance for children was a move toward that utmost of un-American policies, "government medicine." And when SCHIP was up for reauthorization in 2007, the "political stream" had continued its shift to even more partisan polarization (see Abramowitz 2010). Almost all of the northeastern Republicans were gone from Congress, especially the "liberal" Republicans like John Chafee and James Jeffords.[61] Chafee died in 1999; Jeffords became an independent in 2001 and caucused with the Democrats before retiring from the Senate in 2006. There was no replacement for Chafee within a Republican Party that was continuing to move to the right.[62] Chafee was deeply committed to expanding health benefits for children and the disabled through the Medicaid program and was very influential in the Senate on health issues (see Smith 2002: 63–66).

Notes

1. Advisory, Subcomm. on Health of the H. Comm. on Ways and Means, 105th Cong. (March 20, 1997).

2. The number of 10.5 million uninsured children included the 1 million fourteen- to eighteen-year-olds whose Medicaid coverage was to be phased in by 2002 (Nather 1997a).

3. Some sources suggested that Clinton's health proposals were intended to restore the credibility with children's advocates that he lost with his support of the Personal Responsibility and Work Opportunity Reconciliation Act of 1996 (Serafini 1997).

4. This committee was called the Committee on Energy and Commerce from 1981 to 1994, named the Committee on Commerce from 1995 to 2000 during the time that SCHIP was enacted, and in 2001, again named the Energy and Commerce Committee.

5. The Commerce Committee had (as does Energy and Commerce) jurisdiction over the Medicaid program, as well as public health programs. This committee shares jurisdiction over Part B of Medicare, which funds outpatient services, with the Ways and Means Committee, which has jurisdiction over health programs funded by payroll taxes. Ways and Means has sole jurisdiction over Medicare Part A, which pays for hospital care.

6. Bill Thomas (R-CA), the chair of the Health Subcommittee of the Ways and Means Committee, proposed that the $16 billion for children's health in the budget agreement, discussed next in this chapter, be spent on tax deductions for parents who purchase health insurance. Such a provision would fall within the jurisdiction of Ways and Means as a tax measure. At the same time, Thomas Bliley Jr. (R-VA), the chair of the Commerce Committee, also claimed jurisdiction, with a proposal to use the $16 billion for Medicaid expansion (Nather 1997d).

7. The committee, however, rejected by 11–9 an amendment sponsored by Senator Hatch to increase the tobacco tax still further and add $20 billion (Nather 1997f). A week later on the Senate floor, Senator Kennedy sponsored an amendment (cosponsored by Senate minority leader Daschle) to increase the tobacco tax by $.23 per pack and increase spending for children's health insurance by another $12 billion. Kennedy argued that in order to cover all 10.5 million uninsured children, it was necessary to fund the program at $36 billion for five years. Interestingly, Senator Hatch voted against the amendment, while the White House, in a reversal of its earlier position, supported it. The amendment was decisively defeated 30–70 (Nather 1997g).

8. Interview, White House staff, May 10, 1999; interview, House Democratic staff #1, May 12, 1999; interview, House Republican staff #2, May 10, 1999.

9. Interview, House Republican staff #2, May 10, 1999.

10. In an essay originally written in 1977 about the prospects for national health insurance, Theodore R. Marmor (1983) argued that the characteristics of children's health care (its preventive and routine nature, its effectiveness, and

its relative inexpensiveness) would make a plan for universal health insurance for pregnant women and children a promising incremental strategy for achieving national health insurance.

11. *Health Insurance for Pregnant Women and Children: Hearing Before the Subcomm. on Health of the H. Comm. on Ways and Means*, 101st Cong. (March 20, 1990).

12. Theda Skocpol argues that the right wing of the Republican Party, led by conservative intellectuals like William Kristol, saw in the defeat of the Clinton plan an opportunity to attack liberalism in general and generate support for the dismantling of other liberal programs (Skocpol 1997).

13. The Mitchell plan included federal subsidies for premiums for people with low incomes, but provided that pregnant women and children would be eligible for premium assistance at higher income levels. It also included EPSDT-type benefits for children and required that coverage for children and women be the last to be eliminated if program cutbacks were made (CDF memo, August 12, 1994). Senator Christopher J. Dodd offered an amendment that required that all pregnant women and children have insurance coverage by 1995 rather than in 1997 as required in the Mitchell bill. This amendment was approved by the Senate in a 55–42 vote (Rubin and Cloud 1994).

14. The Harkin plan also provided for long-term benefits for at-home or community care for the disabled and the elderly, tax deductions for health insurance purchased by the self-employed, and anti-fraud efforts (Harkin 1994).

15. Children First, "Dear Colleague" letter, September 21, 1994.

16. A policy team within the administration (including staff from the White House, Department of Health and Human Services, and Office of Management and Budget) had also begun to work on incremental health reform proposals as it became clear that national health reform was problematic. Covering uninsured children was one of the major options discussed. White House staff worked with Senate staff on the children's health insurance bill proposed in August 1994 (interview, Clinton White House Staff, May 12, 1999).

17. "Health Coverage for All Children," Office of Senator Kerry.

18. Interview, Senate Democratic staff #4, January 13, 1999.

19. Interview, Families USA staff #1, January 12, 1999.

20. Interview, Senate Democratic staff #3, February 25, 1999.

21. Interview, Families USA staff #1, January 12, 1999.

22. Interview, House Republican staff #2, May 10, 1999.

23. *Governors' Perspective on Medicaid: Hearing Before the S. Comm. on Finance*, 105th Congress (March 11, 1997).

24. See Thompson (1998) for a summary of the complicated judicial and administrative history of this Medicaid payment provision.

25. *Governors' Perspective on Medicaid*.

26. Interview, Senate Democratic staff #5, November 5, 1998; interview, Senate Republican staff #2, February 25, 1999.

27. Interview, Senate Republican staff #4, May 12, 1999.

28. Interview, House Republican staff #2, May 10, 1999.

29. Interview, NGA staff #1, November 6, 1998.

30. *Children's Access to Health Coverage: Hearing Before the Subcomm. on Health of the H. Comm. on Ways and Means*, 105th Congress (April 8, 1997).

31. Ibid., p. 65.

32. Interview, House Republican staff #1, May 11, 1999.

33. Interview, NGA staff #1, November 6, 1998.

34. Interview, House Democratic staff #1, May 12, 1999.

35. Kennedy office memo, May 23, 1996.

36. Kennedy office staff memos, May 23, 1996; October 10, 1996; November 22, 1996.

37. Interview, CDF staff #2, February 25, 1999.

38. Interview, CDF staff #3, June 18, 1999.

39. Kennedy office staff memo, November 22, 1996.

40. Interview, Senate Democratic staff #1, November 6, 1998; interview, Senate Democratic staff #2, October 20, 1998.

41. Interview, Senate Democratic staff #1, November 6, 1998.

42. The Kerry-Kennedy bill and the Hatch-Kennedy bill differed in two other important ways. The former would have expanded coverage for pregnant women, while the latter did not. A Kennedy staff member attributed this to a very high cost estimate for the inclusion of pregnant women and a lack of data about just how many pregnant women remained uninsured following Medicaid expansions (interview, Senate Democratic staff #2, October 20, 1998). In addition, the Kerry-Kennedy bill had no language restricting coverage of immigrants, while the Hatch-Kennedy bill followed the restrictions in 1996 legislation, which prohibited legal immigrants from receiving any public benefits until they had been present in the United States for five years (interview, Senate Democratic staff #1, November 6, 1998).

43. Interview, Senate Democratic staff #1, November 6, 1998; interview, Senate Republican staff #1, November 6, 1998.

44. Interview, Senate Democratic staff #2, October 20, 1998.

45. Interview, Senate Democratic staff #1, November 6, 1998.

46. Interview, Senate Democratic staff #2, October 20, 1998.

47. Interview, House Republican staff #2, May 10, 1999.

48. Interview, Senate Republican staff #1, November 6, 1998.

49. Ibid.

50. Ibid.

51. Interview, House Republican staff # 1, May 11, 1999.

52. *Children's Access to Health Coverage*, p. 36.

53. Ibid., p. 37.

54. Interview, House Republican staff #1, May 11, 1999.

55. Statement of Senator Edward M. Kennedy, Introduction of Family Values Child Health Insurance Act, n.d.

56. Remarks by Senator Hatch, March 13, 1997.

57. Interview, CDF staff #3, June 18, 1999.

58. Ibid. The children's advocacy and health advocacy groups and professional and trade associations that supported the Medicaid eligibility expansions

and opposed the Medicaid block grant also mobilized their members in support of the Senate over the House bill. Senators Rockefeller and Chafee joined with outside advocates to support the Senate bill in the conference committee (Nather 1997h).

59. Interview, CDF staff #3, June 18, 1999.

60. Interview, Senate Republican staff #2, February 25, 1999.

61. Based on a composite score of votes on social, economic, and foreign policy issues, Chafee was the most liberal Republican in the Senate during the 105th Congress (Cohen 1998).

62. His son Lincoln Chafee was appointed to his seat and then elected to the Senate for one term, but he lost to a Democrat in 2006. Lincoln Chafee then became a successful independent candidate for governor of Rhode Island.

4

Ideological Conflict over a "Bipartisan" Program

When it was created in 1997, the State Children's Health Insurance Program (SCHIP) was authorized for ten years, so on September 30, 2007, it was due to expire. Despite its reputation as a bipartisan, popular program, it was not reauthorized in 2007 or 2008. President George W. Bush and the Democratic majority in Congress profoundly disagreed about the future of the program. Democrats wanted to use the reauthorization process to expand SCHIP by increasing the funding for the program, raising the eligibility level, and including new benefits. In fact, key health policy leaders in the House said that an expansion of children's health insurance would be "the signature Democratic health achievement" of the 110th Congress (quoted in Pear 2007). In contrast, President Bush, congressional Republicans, and conservative think tanks described the expansion of SCHIP as an action that would breach the boundary between a private, market-based health-care system and a public one. The president's assistant for economic policy said that it would "move the nation towards 'a single-payer health care system with rationing and price controls'" (Pear 2007). These opponents viewed SCHIP expansion as a foreshadowing of the debate over expanding health coverage to all. In 2007, the president twice vetoed reauthorizing legislation passed by Congress.

Some of the issues of contention, such as the opposition of Republicans to states' use of federal SCHIP funding to cover uninsured adults, were resolved during the 2007 congressional committee negotiations. Yet, President Bush's vetoes of the expanded SCHIP legislation and the failure of advocates for SCHIP reauthorization to get enough support from House Republicans to override the vetoes, resulted in a stalemate on SCHIP while Bush was in office. Both sides linked children's health coverage to the broader issue of universal coverage and health system reform. The expansion and reauthorization of the children's health insurance program happened only after a Democratic president with an enlarged Democratic congressional majority was inaugurated in January 2009. These events are an echo of events in the 1950s and 1960s, when failed efforts to enact a hospital insurance program for the elderly (Medicare) did not succeed until Lyndon Baines Johnson was elected president along with a large majority of liberal Democratic members of Congress.

Within this chapter, I will first describe the contested policy issues debated during the consideration of SCHIP reauthorization and then the related legislative and executive actions. These include the passage of reauthorizing legislation in the House and Senate three times, two presidential vetoes, regulatory action by the Bush administration designed to limit SCHIP expansion, and the response of states and members of Congress to this administrative action. I then discuss the policy outcomes—program changes and innovations that were included in the 2009 reauthorizing legislation, the Children's Health Insurance Program Reauthorization Act of 2009 (CHIPRA). Here, as in Chapter 3, I am examining the relationships between policy process and outcomes.

SCHIP at Ten: Reauthorization Issues

As discussed in Chapter 3, state governors, particularly Republican governors, worked very closely with the Republican congressional leadership in 1997 to create a vehicle for children's health insurance that was not an "entitlement program." SCHIP gave states autonomy in decisions about program structure, eligibility, and benefits. As of 2007, eighteen states had created separate SCHIP programs, ten states and the District of Columbia used SCHIP funding to expand Medicaid coverage, and twenty-two states used federal money for both purposes (Mann 2007). During the ten years of the program's existence, some states had used their SCHIP money to cover parents of children in the program, to cover families with higher incomes than the federal minimum, and even to cover childless adults. The 2007–2008 policy discussions about the reauthorization of SCHIP included proposals to continue and even expand these types of state options and other proposals to prohibit the inclusion of these groups in future SCHIP coverage.

A major accomplishment of the State Children's Health Insurance Program was the reduction of the number of uninsured children in the United States. As discussed in Chapter 3, the 1997 legislation provided that states could use federal money to cover children in families with incomes up to 200 percent of the federal poverty level (FPL) or 50 percentage points above the state's prior Medicaid income level. (According to the Federal Register, in 1997, the federal poverty level for a family of three was an income of $13,330; for a family of four it was $16,050.) In 1997, only three states provided health coverage for such children; as of July 2006, forty-one states and the District of Columbia did so. As medical costs increased, fewer employers provided affordable health insurance to their employees and their dependents. While the number of uninsured adults increased in the period between 1997 and 2005, the proportion of low-income children without health insurance declined by one-third (Mann 2007).

The outreach provisions of the SCHIP legislation also helped to increase the number of children covered by Medicaid. States simplified the application and enrollment processes for SCHIP and Medicaid and mounted outreach and enrollment efforts involving a wide variety of community institutions. The Clinton administration made outreach a priority, pushing both federal agencies and the states in the effort. Corporations and foundations, notably the Robert Wood Johnson Foundation, made major contributions as well (Thompson 2012: ch. 3). In addition to providing coverage to 6 million children through SCHIP, another 6 million children were added to the Medicaid program. However, when SCHIP came up for reauthorization, there were still 9 million uninsured children in the United States. Most (87 percent) of these children were eligible for SCHIP or Medicaid but not enrolled (Mann 2007).

Different policy actors held different views on which reauthorization issues were of greatest importance. These issues also varied as to the level of conflict or consensus that they evoked. In the next several pages I will briefly describe the major issues that were debated during the SCHIP reauthorization process, with the more controversial issues first.

Program Scope: Level of Funding and Eligibility

In his fiscal year 2008 budget proposal (issued in February 2007), President Bush included $4.8 billion over five years for SCHIP and stated that SCHIP coverage should be limited to uninsured children in families with incomes below 200 percent of the FPL. The administration believed that expanding coverage to children in families with higher incomes would result in "crowd-out," the substitution of public coverage for private coverage (BNA 2007d), and that this would weaken the private insurance system. In the president's view, health insurance coverage for children in families with incomes above 200 percent of the FPL should be purchased by their families via tax credits or other mechanisms within the tax code (Teske 2007d). President Bush had previously proposed several changes in tax policy that would encourage the expansion of health savings accounts (BNA 2006b). Thus, the administration was setting the "boundaries" between the "public" and "private" health-care sectors at 200 percent of the FPL. In August 2007, after Congress had passed bills that raised the income eligibility level for SCHIP, the Bush administration sent a letter to the states mandating that they carry out a series of strategies to prevent crowd-out, before they would be allowed to include children in families with incomes above 250 percent of the FPL in their state programs. There was tremendous negative response to this action, which will be discussed later in this chapter.

The administration's position was not supported by either major health industry groups or groups representing other large corporations. Instead, its allies on SCHIP reauthorization were Republican members of Congress and conservative think tanks and interest groups. For example, a May 22, 2007, policy statement issued by thirty-seven health policy experts convened by the Galen Institute, the Heritage Foundation, and the American Enterprise Institute urged Congress to enact President Bush's SCHIP reauthorization plan and stated that families with incomes above 200 percent of the FPL should purchase private health insurance with the help of federal vouchers and tax credits (Teske 2007a). At a February 2007 hearing of the Health Subcommittee of the House Energy and Commerce Committee, Nina Owcharenko, a senior policy analyst at the Heritage Foundation's Center for Health Policy Studies made the same argument. "Reforms" to the tax system, she said, would allow families with incomes above 200 percent of the FPL to buy their preferred type of health insurance coverage, including across state borders (Owcharenko 2007). A number of conservative "tax-payer" groups (including Americans for Tax Reform, Americans for Prosperity, and the National Taxpayers Union) wrote to Republican Senate Finance Committee members Charles Grassley and Orrin Hatch asking them not to raise the federal tobacco tax and not to expand SCHIP: "Instead of morphing the (SCHIP) program into a universal entitlement, we . . . urge you to *seek free market reforms to empower low-income working families* and strengthen access to private health care coverage. . . . Expansion of the program is the wrong direction" (quoted in BNA 2007d, emphasis added).

In contrast to the Bush administration, congressional Democrats, children's advocacy groups, and liberal policy experts believed that the program's funding should be expanded and should allow states to cover children in families with incomes considerably higher than 200 percent of the FPL. Cindy Mann, the executive director of the Center for Children and Families at the Georgetown University Health Policy Institute, suggested in 2007 testimony to the Senate Finance Committee that the most important reauthorization issues were raising the level of program funding and finding ways to overcome the barriers to enrollment. The $5 billion allocated for SCHIP in 2007 was, she noted, not even enough for states to continue covering already enrolled children (Mann 2007; see BNA 2006f). The various bills introduced by Democratic Senate and House members in 2007 would allocate an additional $35 billion to $50 billion to the program over a five-year period and would allow states to cover children in families with incomes at least to 300 percent of the FPL. A bill introduced by Senator Hillary Rodham Clinton and Congressman John Dingell would cover children in families up to 400 percent of the FPL (Committee on Energy and Commerce 2007).

Republicans often evoked the evil of crowd-out during the SCHIP reauthorization debate. But there was disagreement in the health policy literature about the extent to which crowd-out occurred (and would occur under various conditions), the causal direction of the relationship between decreasing private coverage and increasing public coverage, and most importantly, whether this phenomenon should be a major concern. Underlying these disagreements in the literature were differences in basic ideological assumptions about publicly funded health insurance for children.

The Heritage Foundation issued many of their WebMemos during this period on the subject of crowd-out, arguing that expanding SCHIP eligibility to include children in families with higher incomes would encourage parents to leave their private coverage and increase the cost to the taxpayers of covering uninsured children (Heritage Foundation

2007a, 2007b). However, the studies that these reports discuss do not demonstrate the direction of causal relationships between projected reductions in the proportion of children covered by private insurance and increases in children covered by public insurance. It is not clear, for example, whether employees who chose not to pay premiums for their children's insurance under their employer's plan did so because of the existence of SCHIP or would have refused it in any case.

In contrast, studies from centrist and liberal think tanks found less crowd-out and suggest that the issue is the affordability of premiums. One congressionally mandated study of ten states (a study that actually surveyed parents of enrolled children rather than estimating enrollment trends) found that only 14 percent of children who were enrolled in SCHIP in 2007 had been covered by private insurance during the previous six months and that half of their parents said that they could not afford the premiums (Sommers et al. 2007; see also Zuckerman and Perry 2007). The Congressional Budget Office found that the limited data available suggested that parents may choose to drop private coverage because of the greater affordability or superior benefits in the public insurance options that they have (Iglehart 2007a). But to reiterate, because this was such a key concept during the debate, whether or not this phenomenon is viewed as *problematic* depends on the viewer's ideological position on public coverage. I will come back to this issue in Chapter 5 when I discuss the framing of SCHIP expansion.

Adult Coverage

Another issue on which there was disagreement along party lines was that of adult coverage. Fifteen states covered parents, pregnant women, and even childless adults with SCHIP funding, and Republicans were critical of this. Congressman Michael C. Burgess (R-TX) introduced legislation into the House in February 2007 that would end state waivers for the purpose of covering nonpregnant adults under SCHIP and prohibit such waivers in the future (Richmond 2007c). At a Senate Finance Committee hearing on February 1, Senator Charles Grassley famously said, "I fear that using these limited federal dollars for adults has undermined the coverage of low income children. The SCHIP program is for kids. The C stands for children. There is no 'A' in SCHIP."[1] This statement, "there is no A in SCHIP," was heard very often by the advocates for SCHIP expansion during their visits to the offices of congressional Republicans.[2] Governor Sonny Perdue of Georgia, representing the Southern Governors Association at this Finance Committee hearing, framed it as an equality issue. While some states covered adults, he said, others, like Georgia, found it difficult to find enough money to cover all of the low-income children residing within their borders.

In contrast, Democratic Finance Committee chairman Max Baucus referred to research that found that parental coverage was linked to the likelihood that their children would be enrolled and remain in SCHIP. This was an argument for parental coverage often used by Democrats in the House as well (Richmond 2007c). Although the position of the Republican members of the Senate Finance Committee was that SCHIP was a program for children and that adults should not be covered, the exception that came to be made was for pregnant women.

Coverage of Pregnant Women

As part of the Medicaid expansions of the 1980s, Medicaid coverage was mandated for pregnant women with incomes below 133 percent of the FPL and was a state option for women with incomes up to 185 percent of the FPL. As discussed in Chapter 2, the expansion of Medicaid coverage for pregnant women was framed as a solution to the problem of the relatively high US infant mortality rate. When SCHIP was enacted in 1997, pregnant women were not included in the program. However, during both the Clinton and Bush administrations, executive actions by the Centers for Medicare and Medicaid Services (CMS), the federal agency that administers these programs, provided ways in which states could cover pregnant women and be reimbursed by the federal government at the SCHIP rate, which was higher than the Medicaid rate.

In 2000, the Clinton administration wrote regulations that allowed states to apply for waivers to cover parents and pregnant women under SCHIP, but required children to be covered first. Six states used this waiver process to cover pregnant women. And in 2002 the Bush administration revised the definition of "child" to begin at conception, so that states could provide pregnancy-related services to women, although not health services unrelated to pregnancy. By 2009, fifteen states used this route to cover pregnant women under SCHIP.

According to both congressional staff and the staff of other interest groups, the March of Dimes was a vigorous and effective advocate for inclusion of pregnant women in SCHIP. A consensus on the coverage of pregnant women was achieved "pretty early on" in the Finance Committee process, and although "nothing was noncontroversial . . . it was one of the least contentious issues."[3] Although agreement on coverage for pregnant women in general was reached relatively easily, a very contentious issue was the enrollment of legal immigrant children and pregnant women in SCHIP.

Coverage of Legal Immigrants

One of the provisions of the Personal Responsibility and Work Opportunity Reconciliation Act of 1996 (PL 104-93), the legislation that restructured the public assistance or "welfare" program, prohibited the participation of legal immigrants in any public benefit program until they had resided in the United States for five years. Health coverage under SCHIP was considered to be a public benefit. However, by 2003, twenty states provided health insurance coverage for low-income legal immigrants by using state funds. Almost from the time that this provision was enacted in 1996, the National Council of La Raza, the National Immigration Law Center, and other immigrant advocacy groups worked in coalition with other groups to attempt to reverse it. Organizations supportive of SCHIP coverage for legal immigrant children and pregnant women without the five-year waiting period included the National Governors Association, the National Council of State Legislatures, the American Academy of Pediatrics, Catholic Charities USA, and the March of Dimes (National Immigration Law Center 2007).

Republican members of Congress strongly opposed the enrollment of legal immigrant children and pregnant women in SCHIP before the expiration of the five-year waiting period, while many Democratic members of Congress supported it. However, the very broad and controversial attempt at general reform of US immigration laws, led by President Bush and Senator Edward Kennedy, was occurring just as SCHIP reauthorization was being considered. Its ultimate failure in the Senate was due to opposition by Democrats as well as Republicans (Pear and Hulse 2007), and this made the Democratic leadership hesitant to embrace this issue.

"Shortfalls" and the Funding Formulas

The 1997 SCHIP legislation provided for specific funding allocations to each state based on the state's proportion of low-income, uninsured children (according to census data). But any state that had not used its funds at the end of three years would have those funds redistributed to other states. In the early years of the program, many states did not spend all of their funds within the three years because they were creating enrollment systems, but in later years some states found themselves unable to pay for all of the children that they had enrolled (BNA 2006c). Throughout the history of the program, Congress took short-term actions to address this issue by redirecting unspent SCHIP funds to states that needed it and sometimes appropriating new monies for this purpose (see BNA 2006a, 2006f).

The formula for federal allocations to the states was a key reauthorization issue for governors and state health and budget officials who viewed it as critical to the future fiscal health of their states (BNA 2006a). At a hearing of the Health Subcommittee of the Senate Finance Committee in November 2006, state funding shortfalls were identified as a major barrier to children's coverage by state Medicaid officials, academic researchers, and senators Jay Rockefeller and Orrin Hatch (BNA 2006e). Officials in the states that had lower numbers of uninsured children argued that this was because they had been successful in improving coverage and were disadvantaged by the existing allocation formula (Richmond 2006).

The NGA called for changes in the funding formulas that reflected current state expenditures, enrollment, and population growth so that those states that increased enrollment would not be penalized (BNA 2007c). At the first Senate Finance Committee hearing on SCHIP in 2007, there was bipartisan consensus that the funding formula for allocating money to the states needed to be changed (Richmond 2007b). Along with the state funding formula and the coverage of pregnant women, there was also bipartisan agreement on another issue, the need for further state activity to encourage the enrollment of eligible children.

Outreach and Enrollment

Republicans and Democrats shared a concern that almost three-quarters of the 9 million still uninsured children were actually eligible for SCHIP or Medicaid (Richmond 2007a). Senator Hatch, a Finance Committee member and one of the "fathers of SCHIP" said the enrollment of these children was a "first priority" in SCHIP reauthorization, and along with Democrats and children's advocacy groups, supported expanded outreach efforts (BNA 2007a). As congressional committees discussed reauthorization, liberal think tanks (the Center for Children and Families at Georgetown University, Urban Institute, and Economic and Social Research Institute) issued reports calling for automatic enrollment of children in SCHIP based on their eligibility for other public programs, such as school lunch programs or the Women, Infants, and

Children (WIC) program. Such "express lane eligibility," it was argued, would expand coverage and make it less likely that children would move in and out of coverage (BNA 2006d).

Although both Republicans and Democrats supported increased outreach and enrollment efforts, Republicans wanted these efforts primarily targeted at children in the lowest-income families, and argued that children in higher-income families should not be enrolled in the program until a larger proportion of lower-income children were enrolled.

In addition to the contentious issues about who should be covered by the SCHIP program (in terms of family income, length of time in the United States, and age) and the more consensual issues of state allocation formulas and outreach efforts, the SCHIP legislation became a venue for the consideration of other issues of concern to members of Congress and interest groups. One of these issues was coverage for dental care. Under the 1997 SCHIP legislation, dental coverage was a state option. Although most states had some kind of dental benefit, some had annual financial caps on their benefits and coverage was "unstable" because states could drop or reduce the dental benefits provided (Children's Dental Health Project 2010). Advocates for increased access to dental care wanted to have dental coverage included as a federally mandated benefit in SCHIP. I will discuss this effort, along with the efforts of other advocates for specific benefits and coverage, in Chapter 5.

The Legislative Process in 2007

During the first half of his second term in office, President George W. Bush had a Republican Congress (the 109th) but in 2006, the Democrats won a majority in both Houses of Congress.[4] Right after the election, the Democrats in the House announced that improving federal healthcare programs, including the reauthorization of SCHIP, would be major items on their agenda (Teske 2006b). In December, children's health advocates (the Center for Children and Families at the Georgetown University Health Policy Institute, the March of Dimes, the American Academy of Pediatrics, and the National Association of Children's Hospitals) held a press briefing during which they asked for swift reauthorization of SCHIP and laid out general principles for the legislation. These were increased funding to insure that no child lost coverage, no cuts in Medicaid, incentives to states to make the enrollment process easier, coverage of pregnant women, and the creation of quality measures for children's health care.

However, action on these issues could not be assured, because the president was opposed to the policy direction in which Democrats hoped to move, and the Democratic majority, especially in the Senate, was very small (Teske 2006a). In the House, Democrats were about fifty seats short of the two-thirds vote needed to override a presidential veto. On May 17, Congress enacted $50 billion for SCHIP reauthorization as part of a fiscal year 2008 budget resolution (BNA 2007b), more than twice as much as the $5 billion annually proposed by the Bush administration (Teske 2007a). In July, Senator Max Baucus and Congressman John Dingell (D-MI), the chairs of the Senate Finance Committee and the House Energy and Commerce Committee, introduced bills that provided $35 billion and $50 billion, respectively, in "new" funding for children's health insurance.

Committee Debates

The Senate Finance Committee, which historically has had a culture of bipartisanship, was the venue in which many of the key SCHIP issues were debated and resolved. The Senate version of the first SCHIP reauthorization bill was the result of negotiations among four members of the committee—Chairman Max Baucus; Charles Grassley (R-IA), the ranking Republican member of the committee; and Jay Rockefeller and Orrin Hatch. Senators Hatch and Grassley saw their roles on the Finance Committee as mediators between Republican senators who were less supportive of the program than they were and the Democrats on Finance who wanted a far greater expansion of the program. One Republican staff member noted, "Grassley and Hatch wanted the majority of the caucus to be with them. It was very important for Finance on the floor that the majority of Republicans were comfortable with the deal."[5] Grassley and Hatch wanted SCHIP to insure that all low-income children had health insurance and thus supported expanded program funding, in opposition to the administration's position. At the same time they strongly believed that federal funding should not be used to cover either children in higher-income families or adults.

Within the Senate Finance Committee, there was debate about the level of income eligibility. Republicans, and some Democrats, such as Senator Kent Conrad of North Dakota, believed that eligibility of up to 300 percent of the FPL was too high. According to Senator Conrad, the program should only cover children with "low to moderate family incomes." Senator Trent Lott (R-MS) told reporters it is "absolutely outrageous" that the CMS had granted waivers for children in higher-income families (quoted in Teske 2007b).

In early July, the Senate Finance Committee reached a tentative bipartisan agreement to authorize $35 billion for SCHIP and fund it with a $.61 increase in the tobacco tax. On July 10, President Bush said that he would "resist Congress's attempt to federalize medicine" (quoted in Teske 2007c). In a joint statement on July 12, Grassley and Hatch criticized Bush for threatening a veto and said that they had been trying to "hold the line" in the Finance Committee negotiations to keep the cost of SCHIP as low as possible and to prevent new mandates. Without negotiations, they said, a Democratic bill would continue "all the terrible policy provisions that have evolved, such as waivers for childless adults and coverage for higher income kids." In addition to criticizing Bush for his veto threats, senators Grassley, Hatch, and Pat Roberts (R-KS) sent a letter to the president and Department of Health and Human Services (DHHS) secretary Michael O. Leavitt asking them to stop approving state waivers for the coverage of adults under SCHIP (BNA 2007f).[6] In response to the Senate Finance Committee SCHIP deliberations, Leavitt said, "We do not support a massive expansion of *government-run health care* and higher taxes, as the Senate Finance Committee proposes. . . . We are ready to renew our commitment to low income children today, *but we cannot agree to a gradual government take-over of health care—and neither will the American people*" (quoted in Teske 2007d, emphasis added).

The issue of covering legal immigrant children and pregnant women was a contentious one in the Senate Finance Committee in 2007; both Republicans and conservative Democrats were opposed to lifting the five-year ban.[7] Senators Grassley and Hatch, both opposed to ending the waiting period, were very active on this issue in the committee.[8] Senate Democrats also debated this issue internally;[9] they did not want to force their members to take an "immigrant vote" in a period in which immigration was a highly controversial issue.[10] When SCHIP reauthorization was actually enacted in 2009, the larger immigration debate was not as heated.

The SCHIP reauthorization bill approved by the Senate Finance Committee would raise the eligibility for coverage to children in families with incomes up to 300 percent of the FPL; above that income level states would receive less money from the federal government. States would receive lower reimbursement rates for parents who were already in the program, would not be allowed to enroll parents in the future, and would have to phase out coverage for childless adults. Coverage would be extended to 3.2 million additional children. The vote was 17–4 with all the Democrats and six of the Republicans senators (Grassley, Hatch, Roberts, Gordon Smith of Oregon, Mike Crapo of Idaho, and Olympia Snowe of Maine) voting for it (Teske 2007d).

In the House, both the Ways and Means Committee and the Energy and Commerce Committee worked on the SCHIP reauthorization bill, and in both committees there was partisan conflict. In the Ways and Means Committee, much of the conflict related to Democratic proposals to cut $50 billion in Medicare reimbursement to managed care plans (Medicare Advantage) by reimbursing them at the same rates as fee-for-service Medicare providers. In Energy and Commerce, there was opposition from Republicans to the Democratic proposal to raise eligibility levels, which was framed as movement toward "government-run" universal health care. In the words of Congressman Joe Barton (R-TX), the ranking minority member of the committee, "The Democratic bill before us . . . will only end up doing what government-run universal health care systems do best—putting patients in line, rationing care and spreading misery" (quoted in Teske and Plank 2007).

The House and Senate Reauthorization Bills

The House passed the Children's Health and Medicare Protection Act of 2007 (CHAMP Act, HR 3162) on August 1, 2007. The bill authorized $50 billion for five years and was intended to cover an additional 5 million children. Funding for the program was to come from a $.45 increase in the tobacco tax and reductions in payments to private Medicare Advantage plans and other special private Medicare plans (CCF 2007a). This linking of changes in Medicare reimbursement provisions with the SCHIP reauthorization was intended as a way to enact these Medicare cuts in spite of opposition from the managed care industry (Teske 2007f). House Republicans opposed the bill and the 225–204 vote was along party lines. (Five Republicans joined 220 Democrats in voting for it; 10 Democrats and 194 Republicans voted against it.)

The House bill addressed the issues of the allocation of funds to the states, the level of income eligibility, enrollment, crowd-out, coverage of adults, the measurement of quality of care, and dental and mental-health coverage. State allocations were to be calculated on the basis of the actual past use of funds and projected future need; the time that states could use their allotted funds was shortened from three to two years; and a special fund was established for states that experienced a shortfall based on higher than expected enrollment. States that increased enrollment, especially of children in families with the lowest incomes, would receive federal bonuses. Such bonuses would depend on state adoption of a variety of measures that made the application process for coverage and renewal of coverage "user-friendly," including the elimination of face-to-face eligibility interviews, twelve-month continuous eligibility, and the determination of eligibility based on eligibility for other federal programs (express lane eligibility).

The bill also responded to Republican concerns about crowd-out by including a demonstration program in which employers who paid at least 50 percent of the insurance premiums would be able to provide a SCHIP/Medicaid package to their low-income employees. It established a Children's Access, Payment, and Equality Commission to monitor the adequacy of provider reimbursement under SCHIP and Medicaid, and requested that DHHS develop measures of quality for child health services. It also mandated a dental benefit for all enrolled children and parity in mental and physical health benefits.

On issues related to eligibility, the House raised the maximum eligibility age from eighteen to twenty, and gave states the option to include pregnant women in SCHIP without requesting a federal waiver as long as they already covered pregnant women with incomes up to 185 percent of the FPL in their Medicaid program. It allowed states that already covered parents to continue to do so, but phased this out over time and prohibited future coverage of childless adults. The House bill also allowed states to use federal funds to cover legal immigrant pregnant women and children, thus ending the five-year ban on such coverage, but reaffirmed that federal monies could not be used to cover illegal immigrant children (CCF 2007a).

The Senate bill, which was enacted two days after the House bill, authorized $35 billion in additional funding for SCHIP for five years, $15 billion less than the House, and funded it with a higher $.61 increase in the tobacco tax. This difference is because the Senate did not include the savings from the changes in Medicare reimbursement that the House bill did. The Senate bill was similar to the House bill on the issues of the reconfiguration of the state allocation formula,[11] encouraging and simplifying enrollment, a transition period for moving both parents and childless adults out of SCHIP, and child health quality improvements. Like the House bill, it gave states the option to cover pregnant women, and both bills provided a higher matching rate to the states for funds used to provide translation services during the enrollment process. The Senate bill dealt with the issue of a lack of access to dental care, not by mandating dental coverage as the House did, but by providing $200 million in grants to state programs that improved dental coverage for children (CCF 2007b). While they ultimately lost, some Republican members of the Senate opposed the consensus reached among Republican Finance Committee members and Democrats. There were many Republican amendments on the Senate floor and a Republican leadership bill that would fund reauthorization at a total of $9.8 billion over five years (Teske and Hyland 2007).

There were two important areas in which there was a substantial difference between the House and Senate bills. The Senate, but not the House, set an income ceiling for the enhanced federal match for SCHIP at 300 percent of the FPL. If a state chose to cover children in families with higher incomes, it would only receive the lower Medicaid match. (An exception was made for states that already covered children in higher income families.) And the Senate, unlike the House, did not allow states to use federal monies to cover legal immigrant pregnant women and children before they were present in the United States for five years.

As Congress deliberated, President Bush threatened to veto a SCHIP reauthorization bill that expanded program funding and eligibility. After such a bill passed each House, but before negotiations between the houses had concluded, the Bush administration issued regulations with the goal of preventing crowd-out as states enrolled eligible children in SCHIP.

The August 17 Directive

On August 17, 2007, the Centers for Medicare and Medicaid Services sent a letter to state health officials stating that before they could offer health insurance to children in families with incomes above 250 percent of the FPL, they must engage in several strategies for preventing crowd-out. These strategies included verifying the insurance status of applicants via several different databases, preventing employers from dropping children's coverage, requiring premiums that were equal to those imposed with private coverage, and mandating waiting periods of at least one year before children could be enrolled.

In addition, CMS was now requiring that states ensure that the proportion of the population with private health insurance coverage had not decreased by more than 2 percent during the past five years and that *at least 95 percent of children in the state in families with incomes below 250 percent of the FPL* were enrolled in SCHIP before program eligibility could be expanded to those children in families with incomes above 250 percent of the FPL. An official of the National Association of State Medicaid Directors noted that most states do not enroll more than 70 to 85 percent of the children in such families because of factors such as homelessness and limited literacy. This letter was issued late on a Friday afternoon and became known within the child health policy community as "the August 17 directive."

The CMS August 17 directive represents an exquisite irony with regard to the ideological position of the Bush administration. By issuing this directive, it was acting counter to the principles of state autonomy that Republicans had celebrated in the creation of SCHIP. This reversal of state autonomy within the federal system was in service to the principle of maintaining the ideological boundaries of the public and private sectors in the health-care system.

These rules were opposed by the National Association of State Medicaid Directors, health advocacy groups, Democratic members of Congress, the American Public Human Services Association, the governors of New York and California, and forty-four senators from both parties (Teske 2007e; BNA 2007i). On September 12, a group of senators introduced a bill to block the implementation of these new CMS policies (BNA 2007j). The ideological reversal worked both ways. Some of the organizations that argued at SCHIP's creation that too much autonomy was being given to the states were now arguing that the CMS rules were abrogating positive state flexibility in eligibility and benefit decisions. For example, a press release from Families USA stated, "Under current law, states can decide for themselves what the income limit for SCHIP should be. This new policy guts the ability of states to tailor their own SCHIP programs" (Teske 2007e). Opposition to the CMS rules continued during 2008 and will be discussed within that time frame.

The SCHIP Reauthorization Bill

The central issue in negotiations between the House and Senate was whether the Medicare provisions in the House bill should remain as part of the SCHIP reauthorization legislation. The House leadership wanted to continue to link them, but senators Baucus and Grassley, the chair and ranking member of the Finance Committee, respectively, did not (Teske 2007f, 2007g). The major concern of the Democrats in Congress was responding to the threat of the presidential veto. The House and Senate Democratic leadership decided that to minimize this threat, the

House would adopt the Senate bill. While the Senate vote was veto-proof, the House had passed the SCHIP reauthorization bill with less than the two-thirds vote needed for a veto override (Iglehart 2007b).

The final SCHIP bill (The Children's Health Insurance Program Reauthorization Act)[12] was financed through a $.61 rise in the cigarette tax and would provide funding for an additional 4 million children. It contained $100 million in grants for new outreach activities and mandated dental coverage as well as mental-health parity (Teske 2007i). But the five-year ban on legal immigrant access to SCHIP was not changed (as it was in the House bill), and the bill included the Senate's upper income limit of 300 percent of the FPL for SCHIP enrollment under the higher federal match. This bill passed the Senate by 67–29, enough to override the president's veto, but the House vote of 265–159 was not.[13] President Bush had announced that he would veto the bill because of its high cost and because it would increase the federal government's role in health care.

On the Senate floor, Senator Grassley publicly asked the president not to take this action, reminding him of his commitment to lead an effort to provide health insurance to low-income children at the Republican National Convention. He succinctly summarized the arguments made by the president and congressional Republicans opposed to the SCHIP reauthorization bill as he refuted them. He clarified key aspects of the bill that related to Republican concerns: it prevented crowd-out by not allowing states to extend coverage above 300 percent of the FPL without the approval of the secretary of DHHS and unless they meet a target for the percentage of low-income children already covered; it phases adults out of the program; it does not make CHIP an "entitlement," and it "does not make it easier for illegal immigrants to get benefits."[14]

Grassley also chastised the White House and some of his Republican colleagues for the way that they framed the bill, labeling it as "government" or "socialized medicine." It is most interesting to quote his words on this point, words that reflect his commitment to the legislation and frustration with this framing:

> This bill is not a Government take-over of health care, either. And you heard that. This bill is not socialized medicine. Screaming "socialized medicine" during a health care debate is like shouting "fire" in a crowded theatre. It is intended to cause hysteria that diverts people from reading the bill, looking at the facts. To those of you, my colleagues, who make such outlandish accusations, I say: Go shout "fire" somewhere else. Serious people are trying to get real work done. Now is the time to get this work done.[15]

The Presidential Vetoes

President Bush vetoed the Children's Health Insurance Program Reauthorization Act of 2007 on October 3 "because this legislation would move health care in this country in the wrong direction." His criticisms of the bill were that it would allow states to cover children in families with incomes up to almost $83,000 a year, that "government coverage would displace private health insurance for many children," that the bill did not fully fund itself, and that "it raises taxes on working Americans." He repeats the phrase that the bill "moves our health care system in the wrong direction" and says that "our goal should be to move children who have no health insurance to private coverage, not to move children who already have private health insurance coverage to government coverage."[16]

After President Bush vetoed the SCHIP reauthorization bill, senators Grassley and Hatch met with Republican members of the House in an attempt to marshal enough House votes to override the veto. These actions resulted in enmity from the administration and other Republicans. There were policy lunches and meetings where "people were yelling at Senator Grassley and Senator Hatch for working with the Democrats . . . it took a massive amount of political courage to do that."[17]

Before the House vote in response to the presidential veto, advocates contacted House members and held vigils in front of the offices of members of Congress. Groups sponsoring such activity included liberal groups such as MoveOn.org and True Majority and union organizations such as American Federation of Labor and Congress of Industrial Organizations (AFL-CIO); American Federation of State, County, and Municipal Employees (AFSCME); and Service Employees International Union (SEIU). The American Association of Retired Persons (AARP) and the American Medical Association (AMA) were also part of the coalition that sent letters to members of Congress asking them to vote to override Bush's veto (Teske 2007j). Radio and TV ads calling for an override were paid for by the organization representing pharmaceutical companies.[18]

On October 18, 2007, the House failed by thirteen votes to override Bush's veto. All but two Democrats present (229) voted for the override and 44 Republicans did as well. House Republican leaders publicly asked for more negotiations on a new bill; the primary issues were limiting enrollment of children in higher-income families and guaranteeing that no illegal immigrants would be covered (Teske and Nicholson 2007a).

After the failure to override the presidential veto, House Democrats made changes in the bill that they hoped would give them enough Republican support to make it veto-proof. They attempted to respond to Republican concerns about crowd-out, the enrollment of adults, and coverage of illegal immigrant children. The new provisions provided federal funding to the states only for coverage of families with incomes up to 300 percent of the FPL, clarified that federal funds could not be used to include illegal residents in SCHIP, and ended coverage for adults after the first year of the new authorization. It also contained provisions to encourage states to subsidize employer-sponsored health insurance for children as a means to prevent or limit crowd-out and required states to implement other ways to prevent children from leaving employer-sponsored insurance coverage. However, the effort was unsuccessful. HR 3963 was passed by the House on October 25, but the 265–142 vote was less than the two-thirds required to override a presidential veto (Teske and Nicholson 2007b).

While the Senate also approved this bill on November 1, 2007, Democratic and Republican leaders were not able to reach a compromise on legislation that would have gotten enough House Republican votes to override the president's veto. The issues for the Republican House leadership continued to be the inclusion of any adults and the need for guarantees that illegal immigrants and higher-income children would not be eligible for the program (Teske 2007k).

On December 12, President Bush vetoed HR 3963. His second veto message rejected this bill for the same reasons as the first: "It would still include coverage of many individuals with incomes higher than the median income in the United States. It would still result in government health care for approximately 2 million children who already have private coverage." On January 23, the House failed to override the second veto; the vote was 260–152. Congressman John A. Boehner (R-OH), the House minority leader, said that the Democratic SCHIP reauthorization bill would "shortchange low-income children and expand SCHIP coverage to illegal immigrants, adults and those who already have private health insurance" (quoted in Weiland 2008).

About a week after Bush's second veto, Congress passed legislation, almost unanimously,[19] that extended SCHIP through March 2009 and included increased rates for physician payment under Medicare for six months. The legislation did not, however, contain the reductions in

Medicare rates to private managed-care programs that the Democrats had sought and that the Bush administration opposed (Teske 2007l). President Bush signed this bill, HR 3162, the Children's Health and Medicare Protection Act (CHAMP) of 2007.

2008: Responses to the August 17 Directive

In early 2008, Democratic congressional leaders framed the reauthorization of SCHIP as a necessary and important policy response to the loss of jobs and health insurance in a weakening economy (BNA 2008a), but there was little congressional movement on the SCHIP reauthorization during 2008, a presidential election year. There was, however, much activity in response to the administration's August 17 directive to the states limiting enrollment of children in higher-income families unless a set of conditions related to crowd-out were met.

The state of New Jersey filed a lawsuit against DHHS in federal district court in response to the new regulations, claiming that the CMS had violated federal regulatory procedures because it had not had a period of public comments after issuing a regulatory notice. The regulations were also characterized as "arbitrary and capricious." The attorneys general of Connecticut and Massachusetts, the American Academy of Pediatrics–New Jersey, the Office of the Child Advocate of New Jersey, a group of health policy academics, and other advocacy groups all filed amicus briefs in support of the New Jersey action (BNA 2008b). In response to requests from senators Jay Rockefeller and Olympia J. Snowe, both the Government Accountability Office[20] and the Congressional Research Service released legal opinions that the CMS SCHIP directive violated requirements for notification to and review by Congress of agency rulemaking (Teske 2008).

The Health Subcommittee of the Senate Finance Committee held a hearing on the CMS directive on April 9 and the Health Subcommittee of the House Energy and Commerce Committee did the same on May 15. At these hearings, the chairmen of each subcommittee severely criticized the directive (BNA 2008c; Barr 2008a). A group of senators introduced a joint resolution to prevent the CMS August directive from taking effect but then concluded that the time to challenge a regulation under a congressional review procedure had passed (BNA 2008d). This issue was resolved when the Bush administration reversed itself. In August 2008, at the end of the period in which the CMS was to begin enforcement, a CMS spokesman said that the agency was not going to implement the directive (BNA 2008e).

In November 2008, Barack Obama was elected president and Democrats increased their majorities in both houses of Congress. Right after the election, staff of the National Governors Association and state health officials discussed the importance of the reauthorization of SCHIP for state financial planning. Congressman John Dingell (D-MI), chair of the House Energy and Commerce Committee, sent a letter to president-elect Obama discussing the need to act on SCHIP, a first step to broader health reform, as soon as possible (Barr 2008b).

2009: The Enactment of an Expanded Children's Insurance Program

The election of 2008 changed the "political stream," the political environment in which health policy would be made. Democrats now had the presidency and a higher proportion of seats in each House. The number of Democrats in the Senate increased by 8, from 49 to 57, and in the House by 23, from 233 to 256. Many of the concerns of moderate Democrats and Republicans had been addressed during the negotiations over the 2007 legislation, and the expansion of SCHIP had broad support among all sectors of the health-care industry. For the Democrats, the reauthorization of SCHIP, which was only funded through March 2009, was a high priority. And now there was a president who would sign the legislation.

We see again that policy is a result of the interaction of the policy community with the broader political environment. When the 1996 midterm election resulted in conservative Republican control of Congress in 1997, the new children's health insurance program that was created was not a federal entitlement. Similarly, the reauthorization of SCHIP was not possible until the election of 2008 brought a Democratic president to the White House and more Democrats to Congress.

The new House and Senate passed SCHIP reauthorization bills very early in the 111th Congress: the House on January 14 and the Senate on January 29. They were very similar to the legislation that had been passed in 2007. Both included the new allocation formulas to the states and a new process for allocating unspent state funds, both provided states with an option to cover pregnant women without requesting a waiver from DHHS.[21] Both prohibited the coverage of childless adults under SCHIP and future waivers for the enrollment of parents; both reduced the federal match rate for already enrolled parents. The House bill expanded the program to cover an additional 4.1 million children, with funding of an additional $32.3 billion above current program expenses; the Senate funding expansion was $32.8 billion.

Even though the numbers of new Democratic members of Congress assured that the reauthorization legislation would pass, there was still partisan conflict on two major issues: ending the five-year waiting period for legal immigrants and potential crowd-out as the income eligibility level was increased (Barr 2009a, 2009b). In 2009, in contrast to 2007, the Democratic Party was fully supportive of ending the five-year waiting period for the coverage of legal immigrants. According to a Senate staffer who worked on the 2009 reauthorization, there were several reasons for this. In 2009, the general controversy over immigration was "a bit more muted" than it had been in 2007. President Obama had supported the end of this ban when he was a senator, and about half of the states already covered legal immigrant children and pregnant women without the waiting period. The governors in those states voiced their support for its elimination. In addition, the five-year ban was no longer operational with regard to other federal benefits such as the food stamp and school lunch programs.[22]

Politically, it made sense for the Democrats to support benefits for legal immigrants because the votes of Latinas/Latinos were critical to the 2008 election of President Obama and other Democratic candidates. Health care for children was viewed as the least controversial of any issue involving immigrants (Meckler 2009). The children's health advocacy groups that had mobilized support for SCHIP reauthorization in 2007 believed that since Democrats had won the election "we should try to do better . . . that we didn't have to accept what we lost."[23] It was estimated that 400,000 to 600,000 children would be eligible for coverage if the five-year ban was lifted (Pear 2009).

However, while the House bill included the option for states to cover legal immigrant children and pregnant women without the five-year waiting period, and the Senate Finance Committee had approved this provision with a 12–7 vote (a party-line vote with the addition of Senator Snowe), Chairman Baucus's mark did not include this provision. This was because Senator Grassley and other Republicans were still strongly opposed. They argued that ending the five-year ban against legal immigrant children and pregnant women accessing public health insurance coverage would encourage illegal immigration. Senator Grassley had worked so closely with Senator Baucus on so many of the compromises made in 2007 that Baucus did not want to jeopardize Republican support for the whole reauthorization bill. Instead, it was agreed that Senator Rockefeller could introduce an amendment on the Senate floor to eliminate the waiting period for SCHIP coverage for legal immigrant children and pregnant women. Most Senate Republicans were still unhappy with this provision and unsuccessfully fought to exclude it during the amendment process on the Senate floor.[24]

Republicans were also still unhappy about crowd-out and the use of the cigarette tax to finance the program (Iglehart 2009b). Although the Senate Finance Committee chairman's mark included the provision that states would receive a lower matching rate for children in families with incomes above 300 percent of the FPL, Republicans believed that this was not sufficient to prevent crowd-out. In the open executive session of the Senate Finance Committee on January 15, senators Charles Grassley and Pat Roberts (R-KS) described their disappointment that the bipartisan work in 2007 was now nullified. Grassley said that he was "damned disgusted." Senator Roberts said, "We have been thrown underneath the bus."[25] Senators Grassley and Hatch, who had both voted for the 2007 legislation, voted against it in 2009 (Oberlander and Lyons 2009). In their comments on the pending legislation, House Republican leaders said that illegal immigrants would actually be covered, that crowd-out would still occur, and that the tobacco tax was an unstable source of revenue if it encouraged fewer people to smoke (Barr 2009a).

The Children's Health Insurance Program Reauthorization Act of 2009 (CHIPRA) (PL 111-3) authorized $32.4 billion between 2009 and 2013 in addition to annual federal spending of $5 billion a year. It gave states the option to cover children in families with incomes of up to 300 percent of the FPL at the CHIP matching rate. States were allowed to cover children in families with higher incomes, but at the lower Medicaid match rate. The phase-out of adults was contained in the final bill, as was the $.61 increase in the federal cigarette tax. Enrollment performance bonuses to states and "express lane eligibility" were included as new state options in the reauthorizing legislation, but twelve-month eligibility, which had been a state option, was not mandated. DHHS was required to embark on a series of activities to measure the quality of care delivered to children (Iglehart 2009b). Legal immigrant children and pregnant women were finally eligible for health insurance after a decade-and-a-half effort to reverse the 1996 policy decision that excluded them from public benefits for five years after arriving in the United States.

Dental coverage was expanded in the final CHIP reauthorization, including dental coverage for children who have private medical insurance. Preventive dental care and treatment are *mandated* for all children covered by CHIP. States can either establish a set of defined benefits or provide benefits equal to those of one of three benchmark plans (Brooks 2009). Other provisions require that there be an accurate list of dental providers and services on the CHIP hotline and website and that oral health services be included in federal reports on quality of care. A significant Senate floor amendment, sponsored by Senator Snowe, was a provision for "wrap-around" dental benefits for children in families with private insurance. This became part of the legislation. States can provide dental coverage to children who meet the CHIP eligibility requirements, but who have medical insurance with limited or no dental coverage (Children's Dental Health Project 2010).

The reauthorization process was thus used as a "window of opportunity" by advocates for groups such as legal immigrant pregnant women and children and by supporters of expanded benefits such as dental care. In Chapter 5, I will describe the mobilization of groups supportive of the SCHIP expansion and the policy networks concerned about particular issues.

The policy outcome in 2009, once the political stream had shifted, was a substantial expansion of publicly funded children's health insurance. More children were eligible for coverage, there were new mandated benefits, and there were new activities to measure access and quality of care. But these outcomes required major electoral change, because even expanded health insurance coverage for children, one of the populations that most are sympathetic to, was linked to ideological conflict about the nature of the US health-care system. This theme will also be explored in more detail in Chapter 5, where I report on my analysis of the frames used in the policy debate.

Notes

1. Quoted in *The Future of CHIP: Improving the Health of America's Children: Hearing Before the S. Comm. on Fin.*, 110th Cong. (February 1, 2007).
2. Interview, Families USA staff #2, December 2, 2010.
3. Interview, Senate Republican staff #6, December 2, 2010.
4. In the House, the 110th Congress began with 233 Democrats, 198 Republicans, and 4 vacant seats. The Senate was very close with 49 Democrats, 49 Republicans, and 2 independents, one of whom always voted with the Democrats, and the other of whom voted with the Democrats on issues like children's health insurance.

Ideological Conflict over a "Bipartisan" Program   **103**

5. Interview, Senate Republican staff #6, December 2, 2010.

6. In September, Senator Grassley again criticized the president for "drawing lines in the sand" and not being "constructive." Grassley pointed out that if there were an extension of the program instead of a reauthorization, then there would still be adults covered by the program (Teske 2007h).

7. Interview, AAP staff #4, November 11, 2010.

8. Their position was first, that legal immigrants should be taken care of by their official sponsors, and second, that the states that would cover legal immigrants under a provision allowing a disregard of the federal five-year waiting period would be the same states that were already covering them with state funds. (Interview, Senate Republican staff #6, December 2, 2010.)

9. Interview, First Focus staff, December 2, 2010.

10. Interview, Senate Democratic staff #8, December 3, 2010.

11. It, like the House bill, reduced the period of time in which states could use their federal allotment to two years, allocated funds to the states based on need, and set up a contingency fund to pay for additional enrollment.

12. Funding for SCHIP actually expired on September 30, 2007, but a SCHIP funding extension was passed as part of a temporary spending bill for federal agencies through November 16 (Teske 2007i).

13. Forty-five Republicans voted for it, and eight Democrats against it.

14. US Congressional Record, September 26, 2007, S12130.

15. Ibid.

16. GPO Access, Weekly Compilation of Presidential Documents 2007, p. 1298, frwais.access.gpo.gov (DOCID:pd08oc07_txt-15).

17. Interview, Senate Republican staff #6, December 2, 2010.

18. Interview, PhRMA policy staff, December 3, 2010.

19. The legislation was passed by unanimous consent in the Senate on December 18, and by 411–3 in the House.

20. The name of the independent research agency that helps Congress to fulfill its oversight function was changed on July 7, 2004, from the General Accounting Office to the Government Accountability Office.

21. The inclusion of pregnant women in CHIP is a continuation of federal maternal and child health policy over time. From the first federal health legislation (PL 62-116), which established the Children's Bureau in 1912, through the enactment and long history of Title V of the Social Security Act of 1935 (which created the first of a series of grants to the states for maternal and child health programs), the health of children and pregnant women had been legislatively linked, although there have been specific categorical grant programs under Title V that provided funds for services only to children (see Hutchins 1997).

22. Interview, Senate Democratic staff #8, December 3, 2010.

23. Interview, Families USA staff #2, December 2, 2010.

24. Ibid.

25. *Executive Business Meeting to Consider Adoption of the Committee's Rules for the 111th Congress and an Original Bill Reauthorizing the Children's Health Insurance Program: Hearing Before the S. Comm. on Fin.*, 111th Cong. (January 15, 2009).

5

Expanding the Program: Advocacy and Framing

This chapter begins with a description of the interest groups that were active on the reauthorization and expansion of the State Children's Health Insurance Program (SCHIP), and the coalitions and "campaigns" in which they were engaged. I then discuss some of the specific policy networks that used the SCHIP reauthorization process to bring attention to their long-standing concerns. Next, I report on my analysis of the "frames" used by advocates and opponents of program expansion.

Groups, Coalitions, and Advocacy Strategies

SCHIP reauthorization and expansion was supported by a large number of organizations and overlapping coalitions. Groups as diverse as the Children's Defense Fund and the Pharmaceutical Research and Manufacturers of America were part of these coalitions. For several existing policy communities, the congressional imperative to consider reauthorization was a "window of opportunity" to advance specific policies of interest to them.

New Actors on Child Health Policy

In addition to the network of groups and think tanks that had been active on issues related to children's health insurance coverage when

SCHIP was created in 1997 (and in some cases when Medicaid was expanded in the mid-1980s), two new organizations were active on policy research and advocacy related to the SCHIP reauthorization between 2006 and 2009. The first was the Center for Children and Families (CCF) at the Georgetown University Health Policy Institute. This policy research center was established in 2002. Among its supporters are the two major US foundations concerned about expanding health-care access and coverage in general (the Henry J. Kaiser Family Foundation and the Robert Wood Johnson Foundation) and four private foundations concerned with low-income and vulnerable children and families (Anne E. Casey Foundation, David and Lucile Packard Foundation, the George Gund Foundation, and the Atlantic Philanthropies).[1] The second organization, First Focus, is a new children's advocacy group created in 2005.

First Focus was established as an explicitly "bipartisan" national advocacy group, "dedicated to making children and families a priority in federal policy and budget decisions." It presents itself as unique in its bipartisanship and its work to engage the private sector in children's advocacy.[2] First Focus was created by the David and Lucile Packard Foundation and the Atlantic Philanthropies in order to fill what they perceived as a void in children's advocacy at the federal level. While groups concerned with issues of economic equality such as the Center on Budget and Policy Priorities and Families USA were seen as doing excellent advocacy on issues like SCHIP, they were not solely focused on children's issues. And in an era of Republican dominance, the Children's Defense Fund was perceived by these foundations as too politically left to do bipartisan advocacy.

In 2005, these two foundations issued a request for proposal for an existing organization to "incubate" such a bipartisan policy research and advocacy organization. America's Promise Alliance, a child-focused organization created by former general Colin Powell in 1997, received the funding. Initially the organization was called the Children's Investment Fund; in 2006, it was renamed First Focus. Its current president and vice president for health policy came from staff positions in the office of Senator Jeff Bingaman of New Mexico, and both had also worked for health policy interest groups as well as in Congress.

Health is only one of the organization's concerns: it works on a broad range of children's issues, including the environment, education, and poverty. According to a First Focus staff member, "We are still rather small so we are pretty strategic and tactical in terms of our agenda. We still look at the congressional agenda and see where we can exert some influence and move the dial for kids."³ First Focus is a staff rather than a membership organization, but it gives grants to about thirty existing children's health and educational advocacy organizations in key congressional districts. These groups then function as the grassroots in federal advocacy campaigns on children's issues.⁴

The highest priority issue for First Focus in relation to SCHIP reauthorization was improving SCHIP enrollment of eligible children; the organization worked hard to include "express lane" eligibility in the legislation. Other issues of major concern were adding oral health and dental coverage, removing the five-year ban for immigrant pregnant women and children, and including funding for the "nurse-family partnerships" form of home visiting in the SCHIP reauthorization. Both the Center for Children and Families at Georgetown University and First Focus were part of the policy network supportive of the expansion of SCHIP in 2007, and both worked within some of the coalitions that I will next describe.

Advocacy by Supportive Coalitions

One of the major coalitions working on behalf of SCHIP reauthorization included organizations that were part of an informal network called the Children's Health Group. The Children's Health Group began meeting in the offices of the American Academy of Pediatrics (AAP) in 1997 to discuss issues related to children's health-care access.⁵ This network was a descendant of the maternal and child health coalition created by staff at the Children's Defense Fund in the mid-1980s. After the disagreement between CDF and other children's advocacy and health groups over the CDF-Kennedy-Hatch 1997 block grant proposal, CDF moved out of the leadership of the child health coalition and the AAP assumed the role of group convener.

During the most active periods of the debate over SCHIP reauthorization, about sixty groups came together on a weekly basis at the AAP office, including CDF. These were not all children's advocacy groups; the American Association of Retired Persons (AARP) and the American Medical Association (AMA) participated. Included in this coalition were other groups with the capacity to do grassroots mobilization: Families USA, the American Federation of State, County, and Municipal Employees (AFSCME), the Service Employees International Union (SEIU), Voices for America's Children, National Rural Health Association, Acorn, the Center for Community Change, Generations United, Easter Seals, and Community Catalyst.⁶

A smaller group of advocates functioned informally as an executive board to develop strategy for the SCHIP reauthorization campaign. This group included staff from the AAP, March of Dimes, National Association of Children's Hospitals and Related Institutions (NACHRI), the Center for Children and Families, and the Center on Budget and Policy Priorities.[7] These latter two organizations were (and are) primarily policy research organizations; the March of Dimes can be categorized as a "disease" organization; and the AAP and NACHRI are "provider groups."

In December 2006, the CCF issued a policy paper on SCHIP that became the basis for discussions and negotiations about issues such as funding and benefits among groups within the coalition. Once a consensus was reached, all of the groups agreed to endorse joint letters to members of Congress. In addition, a small group met weekly to coordinate media strategy in the effort to get op-eds and letters to the editor published.[8]

Staff of the organizations attending the Children's Health Group meetings would also plan joint visits to members of Congress, which were coordinated by the AAP. There would be a common document outlining the groups' requests on the SCHIP reauthorization, joint "talking points," and then each group involved would discuss their key issue.[9] "The mental-health advocates would talk about mental health, the dental advocates would talk about dental care, and the March of Dimes would talk about pregnant women."[10]

An AAP staff person hired just for this campaign would do a daily e-mail to almost 400 organizations inviting them to participate in scheduled congressional visits. She also mobilized children's advocates in the states to contact their members of Congress with the same messages that were being delivered in Washington, DC. In those states where the AAP chapters were active on policy issues, they usually worked in coalition with child advocacy and other groups. AAP staff viewed the communication of support for SCHIP reauthorization and expansion to members of Congress by such broad state-level coalitions as a very effective advocacy strategy. In the period after the Bush vetoes, the AAP and other groups did more than 100 visits to members of Congress.[11]

While the AAP used its organizational resources to facilitate collective activity on behalf of SCHIP reauthorization, it had its own policy priorities. As noted in Chapter 3, the AAP had sponsored a proposal for universal children's health insurance as early as 1991. In 2007, its focus was on getting as many children covered by the program as politically possible and having a sufficient level of funding to achieve that goal. In addition, AAP members and staff advocated for the development of quality measures for pediatric care (discussed below).

AAP's strategic resources included the respect and authority its members enjoyed on child health issues and the geographic dispersion of its membership. An AAP staff member noted that anecdotes are often more effective than quantitative data in making arguments to members of Congress and that "pediatricians are pretty good about providing anecdotes. They give one or two data points and then they say, 'I have this little Johnny in my office . . . ' and it is a pretty compelling narrative."[12]

While the Children's Health Group took the "lead role" on SCHIP reauthorization,[13] other overlapping coalitions of groups were involved as well. Another informal coalition that worked on the issue of SCHIP reauthorization encompassed groups that had worked together in 1994 and 1995 to oppose the effort of congressional Republicans to transform Medicaid into a block grant to the states (discussed in Chapter 3). After these events, a coalition dedicated to preserving and expanding Medicaid continued to function, facilitated by Families USA. It included hundreds of organizations that met on an ad hoc basis to work on specific Medicaid-related policy issues. Like the Children's Health Group, it had no official structure, membership, or staff. During the SCHIP reauthorization process, groups in both the Medicaid coalition and the Children's Health Group "signed on" to letters written to members of Congress by the other coalition.

As discussed in Chapter 2, the primary mission of Families USA was to act on behalf of low-income people on health-care issues and in the pursuit of full equality in health care. After the failure of the Clinton health-care plan, Families USA, as well as other health advocacy groups, came to view children's health-care coverage as an important incremental step toward universal coverage. It supported the creation of SCHIP and worked with state groups to expand coverage for children at the state level. During the SCHIP reauthorization process, the organization opposed premiums and other forms of cost-sharing for SCHIP and Medicaid recipients. Families USA advocated for twelve months of continuing eligibility and express lane eligibility as federal mandates as well as enrollment performance bonuses to states and continued coverage of adults under SCHIP. It was also very concerned about the overall amount of funding for SCHIP and the formula for the allocation of monies to the states.

Families USA created another coalition in 2006 to focus attention on SCHIP reauthorization: the Campaign for Children's Health. This coalition included many types of organizations: advocacy groups, unions, religious groups, and physician and hospital groups. Many of these groups were already in other children's health coalitions.[14] It was also a partner in "a strange-bedfellows coalition" with the Pharmaceutical Research and Manufacturers of America (PhRMA), the association of large pharmaceutical companies. The executive directors of Families USA and PhRMA met to coordinate advertising and media strategies to support the reauthorization and expansion of SCHIP.[15] In both 2007 and 2009, PhRMA spent millions of dollars on a media campaign, both television and print.[16] And the Bush administration expressed its concerns to the president of PhRMA about this effort (Pear 2007). As the Senate Finance Committee was working on the SCHIP markup in May 2007, a PhRMA print ad said, "America's pharmaceutical research companies strongly support the reauthorization of SCHIP. And we encourage Congress to consider new ways to make SCHIP outreach and enrollment efforts even more effective, ensuring this successful program reaches as many children as possible" (Teske 2007a).

PhRMA's work with Families USA was part of a larger effort by a broad coalition of liberal advocacy groups and organizations representing structural interests in the health-care system (physicians, hospitals, insurers, and the pharmaceutical companies) to work together for health reform focused on expanding coverage. The reauthorization and expansion of SCHIP was a first step in their effort (Starr 2011).

In addition to financing a large media campaign, PhRMA's activity on behalf of SCHIP reauthorization included writing letters to and meeting with members of Congress.[17] In a January 31, 2007, letter to senators Charles Grassley and Max Baucus, Billy Tauzin, the president and chief executive officer of PhRMA (and a former member of Congress), stated,

> PhRMA believes that reauthorizing this critical program should rank high on the agenda of the 110th Congress. . . . We hope that Congress uses the SCHIP reauthorization process not only to extend the program, but also to make outreach and enrollment efforts more effective, to expand opportunities for SCHIP support of employer-sponsored coverage of SCHIP eligible children, and to examine additional opportunities to help ensure that more children receive basic medical treatment and preventive care.[18]

The issues of most importance to PhRMA, in addition to outreach and enrollment, were the expansion of federal funding, premiums for enrollment in employer-sponsored programs, the development of child health quality measures, and support for demonstration programs to reduce childhood obesity. PhRMA did not specifically communicate with policymakers on the provisions covering pregnant women or legal immigrant women and children, or expanded dental coverage, but it advocated for passage of legislation that included these provisions.[19] The significance of PhRMA's support for SCHIP reauthorization and expansion will be discussed later in this chapter as part of my discussion of Republican framing of SCHIP expansion.

Reauthorization as a "Window of Opportunity"

Each of the organizations involved in the SCHIP reauthorization campaign contributed their own unique resources to the effort and each group had certain issues that were of greatest importance to them. These were issues that they had been concerned about for years; the SCHIP reauthorization provided a special opportunity for legislative action.

Pregnant women. One of these issues was coverage of pregnant women under SCHIP. As noted earlier, the March of Dimes, as part of the AAP-facilitated coalition, consistently brought the issue of the inclusion of pregnant women to discussions with members of Congress. Staff of several children's and health-reform advocacy groups, as well as both Democratic and Republican congressional staff, identified the March of Dimes as the major voice for covering pregnant women under SCHIP. The March of Dimes had argued for the inclusion of pregnant women in the original 1997 SCHIP legislation, but the effort was unsuccessful. The March of Dimes "has been a lead forever on this . . . that was their main issue."[20] There was no organized opposition to making it easier for states to include pregnant women in SCHIP, but "a lot of times these provisions don't make it, not because there is opposition, but because no one really cares about it. The March of Dimes worked really hard to make sure that people cared enough to put it in."[21] In the words of the AAP staff member interviewed about SCHIP reauthorization, "Pregnant women, pregnant women, pregnant women—that's what the advocates who would always go with us to these Hill visits would say."[22]

The March of Dimes, as discussed in Chapter 2, has always been regarded as a bipartisan group, one that enjoys positive relationships with both Republicans and Democrats. This is, of course, a major political asset. According to a Republican congressional staff member, the March of Dimes "did some really solid work" on the SCHIP reauthorization; "they were wonderful to work with."[23] When asked about other groups that might have also advocated for coverage of pregnant women, this congressional staffer said that Right to Life groups were "also very supportive on that issue."[24]

Legal immigrants. The issue of ending the five-year ban on public benefits for legal immigrants was also one on which advocacy groups had been active since this ban was enacted in 1996. In 2003, a reversal of the ban was included in Medicare legislation but omitted at the end of conference negotiations (National Immigration Law Center 2007). A Families USA staff member points out, "There was a coalition of groups working on it for a number of years; SCHIP reauthorization just became the place for it to move forward."[25] The National Immigration Law Center (NILC) and the National Council of La Raza (NCLR) were the leaders of this coalition, which included Families USA, the Center for Budget and Policy Priorities, First Focus, and CCF.[26] Staff of the NILC and the NCLR came to the Children's Health Group meetings, and legal immigrant coverage was almost always discussed.[27] Support for the reversal of the five-year ban came from a large number of other groups over the years, including the National Governors Association, the National Conference of State Legislatures, the American Academy of Pediatrics, Catholic Charities USA, the March of Dimes, and hundreds of other liberal and religious organizations (Families USA 2003b).

Quality measurement and delivery models. Another set of issues that was brought into the reauthorization discussion was federal funding for research to develop quality measurements for pediatric health services and studies of SCHIP and Medicaid payment levels. The AAP argued that levels of payment that were far lower than Medicare levels limited pediatrician participation in Medicaid and SCHIP and thus limited access and quality of care for many children. Other groups that joined with the AAP on Capitol Hill in advocating for child health services quality measurement were NACHRI, the March of Dimes, the National Partnership for Women and Families, Families USA, and the Iowa Child and Family Policy Center.[28]

These advocacy efforts were successful. The Children's Health Insurance Program Reauthorization Act (CHIPRA) allocated $225 million from fiscal year 2009 through fiscal year 2013 to the Department of Health and Human Services (DHHS) to establish a program for developing and testing quality child health measures that would evaluate access, stability of coverage, and effectiveness of services in Medicaid and SCHIP. States were required to submit an annual report to DHHS on the quality of child health services, and demonstration grants would be awarded to up to ten states and providers for testing child health measures. CHIPRA also established a Medicaid and CHIP Payment and Access Commission (MACPAC) to evaluate children's access to care and payment policies (CCF 2009). While pediatricians and children's hospitals did not succeed in raising actual reimbursement levels for pediatric services under CHIP and Medicaid, this was achieved with the enactment of the Affordable Care Act in 2010.

Advocacy organizations representing nontraditional health-care delivery models were also successful in getting recognition within CHIPRA. The National Assembly on School-Based Health Care (now the School-Based Health Alliance) together with state-based health center associations had worked for several years to educate members of Congress about the benefits of providing primary care health services to children in schools. CHIPRA provides that states have the option of offering services, "effective immediately," through school-based health centers.[29]

Dental care. The 1997 SCHIP legislation required states that used SCHIP funds to expand their Medicaid programs to provide dental benefits (as part of the Medicaid Early Periodic Screening, Diagnosis, and Treatment benefits), but states that had created a separate SCHIP program were not required to do so. By 2007, there was a great deal of attention to the issue of inequality in access to oral health services in congressional debate over SCHIP reauthorization and policy initiatives that addressed this issue. Beginning in 1997, an outside policy entrepreneur and supportive members of Congress had worked to advance greater access to oral health care, but it was a tragic "focusing event" that brought their work to fruition.

The Children's Dental Health Project (CDHP) was founded in 1997 by Burton L. Edelstein, a pediatric dentist[30] who was a Robert Wood Johnson Foundation fellow in health policy in the Senate office of Senator Tom Daschle in 1996–1997. While Edelstein was working in Congress, SCHIP was created with dental services as only a state option. CDHP's mission was to address the disparities in oral health care and to "represent the oral health interests of children and families in federal and state actions" (*Inside Dentistry* 2011).

CDHP, in coalition with other groups, advocated for a comprehensive approach to improving the access of low-income children to oral health services, including making dental care a mandatory service under SCHIP. Senator Jeff Bingaman (D-NM) and other supportive members of Congress began introducing legislation addressing these issues. Legislation titled the "Children's Dental Health Improvement Act" was introduced by Senator Bingaman into the Senate in 1997, 2001, and 2003, and into the House by Representative John Murtha (D-PA) in 2002 and Representative Michael Simpson (R-ID) in 2004. Aside from a June 2002 hearing held on Bingaman's bill by the Senate Committee on Health, Education, Labor, and Pensions, no action was taken on any of this legislation after referral to a committee.[31]

Between the enactment of SCHIP in 1997 and its reauthorization in 2009, however, federal and state officials, think tanks, and professional dental associations engaged in a series of policy activities that focused attention on the issue of access to oral health care. These included the publication of the Surgeon General's report *Oral Health in America* in 2000, and the publication of reports and congressional briefings by associations of state officials such as the National Governors Association and the National Conference of State Legislators, and think tanks such as the National Health Policy Forum, the Kaiser Family Foundation, the Urban Institute, the Institute of Medicine, the George Washington University Center for Health Policy Research, and the Georgetown University Center on Children and Families.

CDHP organized a coalition of providers, including the American Dental Association, the American Academy of Pediatric Dentistry, the American Dental Hygienists' Association, the National Dental Association, and the Hispanic Dental Association, in a Dental Access Coalition (Edelstein 2009). During the consideration of SCHIP reauthorization in 2007, staff from both the Children's Dental Health Project and the American Dental Association attended meetings of the Children's Health Group. Other groups agreed to include dental benefits as one of the provisions they would ask Congress to include in the reauthorization of the Children's Health Insurance Program (Edelstein 2009).[32]

As mentioned at the very beginning of this book, the "focusing event" that brought the issue of lack of access to routine dental care to the "decision agenda" was the death of Deamonte Driver, a twelve-year-old boy from Prince George's County, Maryland, who died after surgery to treat a brain infection that originated in an infected tooth. Although Deamonte had Medicaid, his mother could not find a dentist who would accept this insurance. When he became ill, the family was living in a homeless shelter and no longer had Medicaid. Deamonte's death was reported in the *Washington Post* and picked up by the national media (Iglehart 2009a).[33]

In response, senators Bingaman and Benjamin L. Cardin (D-MD) introduced the Children's Dental Health Improvement Act of 2007 (S 739) into the Senate on March 1 while Congressman John Dingell introduced companion legislation (HR 17810) into the House on March 29.³⁴ In introducing this bill, Senator Cardin said, "It is outrageous today that in America, a young boy can die because his family can't find a dentist to remove an infected tooth.... Anytime we lose a child, it is a tragedy. But Deamonte Driver's death is particularly devastating because it was easily preventable" (quoted in Otto 2007). Seven other bills to increase children's access to dental care were introduced into Congress in response to Deamonte's death (Edelstein 2009).

On March 27, about a month after the tragedy, the Health Subcommittee of the House Committee on Energy and Commerce held a hearing entitled "Insuring Bright Futures: Improving Access to Dental Care and Providing a Healthy Start for Children." One of the major themes of the hearing was that Deamonte's tragedy was not unique, but that many children without access to dental care were at risk for similar outcomes. Deamonte's name was mentioned twenty-two times during the hearing, and this count does not include several other references to the case of a "twelve-year-old boy from Maryland." Deamonte's death "transformed policymaking on children's oral health by creating a 'face' for the issue ... and crystallized the child health advocacy community around children's oral health" (Edelstein 2009: 470). At the same time, Edelstein argues, this tragic event would not have been as powerful without extensive coverage in the *Washington Post* and the previous years of policy activity by state and local officials, policy research organizations, and health-care provider associations.³⁵

In spite of the discussions of the serious dangers to children from dental disease, much of the framing of the need to expand access to regular oral health care during the March 27 hearing was in terms of the arguments made about children's health care in general: its cost-effectiveness and impact on future productivity. This is analyzed in the next section of this chapter.

Framing SCHIP Expansion

As discussed in Chapter 1, the term *framing* is used to describe the presentation of policy issues in a way that will resonate with shared cultural and political values and thus attract support. Here I report on my examination of the way in which both supporters and opponents of SCHIP expansion used frames that were very similar to frames used in prior policy debates. While advocates for SCHIP expansion were referencing arguments made previously in support of the expansion of public funding for children's health insurance, opponents were framing their opposition in terms used in previous conflicts over general health-system change. The continuity of these themes over time is clearly one way that the concept of "policy legacies" can be made operational. The data used to analyze the framing of SCHIP reauthorization, or more accurately SCHIP expansion, are different for supporters and opponents. Framing by supporters was found primarily in statements by members of Congress, state-level officials, policy experts, and representatives of interest group organizations at congressional hearings. This is because Democrats, the majority party in Congress[36] and supportive of SCHIP expansion, occupied the chairs of committees and controlled the witness list of hearings. In contrast, statements by opponents of SCHIP expansion are found primarily in presidential veto messages and statements by members of the administration and of Congress, but not in congressional hearings.

Framing by Advocates of SCHIP Expansion

A review of both journalistic accounts of the policy debate in 2006–2009 and congressional hearings during that period indicated that advocates for program expansion were using a set of "frames" similar to those used by advocates for the expansion of Medicaid eligibility in the 1980s and the creation of SCHIP in 1997. As discussed in Chapter 2, the frames used in presenting the value of expanding Medicaid eligibility to pregnant women and children in the mid-1980s were (1) the morality of providing care to innocent and vulnerable children, (2) health-care access as an investment in the future US workforce, and (3) the long-term cost-effectiveness of primary and preventive health services for children. During the creation of SCHIP, as discussed in Chapter 3, a fourth frame was used to talk about the "hard-working families" benefiting from the program.

The frames. In order to analyze more systematically which of these frames was used most often, a textual content analysis was conducted. All SCHIP hearings and testimony between 2006 and 2009 that were available electronically were coded, using a set of key words found in statements of elected officials and nongovernmental policy actors.[37]

Each time that one of the key words occurred, the word was highlighted in the text. These word clusters were counted separately for each of the hearings/and or testimony on SCHIP between 2006 and 2009.[38] In addition, as discussed later, each instance of the use of these phrases was then examined to make sure that the phrase was actually part of an argument about the value of children's health insurance.

The first frame that I searched for was that of children as vulnerable and dependent and policy proposals related to caring for children as moral action. The words used to represent this concept were "vulnerable," "vulnerability," "compassion," "compassionate," "moral," and "morality." (This is a frame used in discussing many public policies related to the welfare of children, not just health policy.) This frame is found in the remarks of the Rev. F. Vernon Wright of the Plymouth Congregational Church, United Church of Christ, Helena, Montana, at an April 2007 field hearing of the Senate Finance Committee. He ends his testimony using these words:

> What kind of future are we providing for our children, the future of our Nation, when we allow for millions of American children to be so vulnerable? Truly as a Nation, are we not headed for ship-wreck? I think the moral thing to do is not only reauthorize CHIP, but to act on its expansion, as you stated earlier. In the end, the greatness of our Nation is measured not by our might but by the health and well-being of our peoples and the mercy and *compassion* of our governance.[39] (emphasis added)

This is a clear echo of the framing used by Marian Wright Edelman and the Children's Defense Fund beginning in the early 1980s,[40] but as will be discussed below, this frame was used far less often than the others during the debate over SCHIP reauthorization.

The second frame was the social construction of children eligible for SCHIP as being the children of "working families." This was one of the major frames used by senators Edward Kennedy and Orrin Hatch in discussing their Child Health Insurance and Lower Deficit (CHILD) bill in 1996 and 1997. The terms used to represent this concept were "working families" and "hard-working parents." The "working families" frame is actually explicated by the governor of Montana at the April 2007 field hearing of the Senate Finance Committee.

> Healthy communities start with healthy families, and a healthy start is healthy children. Montana has 13,300 of our children enrolled in the CHIP program that gets the families a healthy start. And some people

> think of the Children's Health Insurance Program *as being intended for indigent families*. It is not. In Montana, 92 percent of the people who are enrolled in the CHIP program have one or both of the *parents working*. These are *working families*, and there is nothing more important to *working families* than a healthy child, because all over Montana there are young families who say a prayer with their children as they tuck them into bed, and after they tuck their children in, they go down the hall and they kneel again and they say a prayer. And this time the prayer is that none of their children gets sick because they do not have health insurance. These are *working families. These are members of our community*.[41] (emphasis added)

In the statement above, we also see an evocation of the dependence and vulnerability of children.

During the same hearing, a divorced and self-employed mother of a child with a seizure disorder tells the story of how the SCHIP program in Montana enabled her son to get treatment. Then she echoes the themes of the governor, emphasizing that the SCHIP program is not just for "low-income people."

> I am not embarrassed to have received these benefits. I am a very *hard-working person,* and I think there is a problem in our society today with American workers, people who are blue-collar workers or people like myself who go out and work *hard every day to pay my fair share of taxes* and then find out I do not have enough money at the end of the day to buy insurance. . . . So I am not embarrassed to accept the benefits that were there in our time of need because to me it is a "hand up."[42] (emphasis added)

The third and fourth frames are future-oriented economic arguments that have been used in previous policy discussions of expanding health insurance coverage for children. One is the "human capital" frame: providing health care to children as a way of investing in their potential as future workers, a necessity for US success in global economic competition. More recently, the ability to learn in school is conceptualized as the intervening variable: children need to be healthy in order to succeed in school and then in the workforce. This concept was labeled as the "education/investment" concept. The words linked to this frame were "learning," "school," "workforce," and "investment."

The other future-oriented economic argument is about the long-term savings derived from providing preventive or primary health care to children. If children have access to primary care, then illnesses or health conditions can be prevented or treated in their early stages and thus money is saved on future health-care costs. It will be recalled that in the 1980s there was the oft-quoted statistic from the Institute of Medicine that $1 invested in prenatal care would save more than $3 in future medical care and social and educational support for a disabled child.[43] The term "cost-effective" was flagged as an indicator of this argument.

Chairman Max Baucus uses both future-oriented economic frames in his opening statement at the February 1, 2007, hearing of the Senate Finance Committee on "The Future of CHIP."

> Children without health insurance are 5 times more likely to have unmet medical needs or to delay necessary care . . . their health and development are at risk. Lack of health insurance can affect school attendance. It can impair a child's ability to grow up healthy and *ready to learn*. Lack of health insurance coverage matters to all Americans. It can lead to a crowded emergency room, it can strain access to care, it can burden our safety net health providers. When care is delayed, diseases that should be easily and *cheaply treated* become major medical crises. Investing in children's health, by contrast, improves our public health, lowers costs, and it will reap a healthy economy for tomorrow's *workforce*.[44] (emphasis added)

In his opening remarks at the "Open Executive Session to Consider the CHIP Reauthorization Act of 2007" on July 19, 2007, he again uses a human capital/future workforce frame. He also refers to the suffering of vulnerable children, but not explicitly to the costs of more complicated care.

> Uninsured children suffer. Uninsured kids are less likely to get care for sore throats, earaches, and asthma. When care is delayed, small problems can become big problems. Nearly half of uninsured children have not had a checkup in the past year. Uninsured children are twice as likely to miss out on doctor visits and checkups. CHIP makes sense as an *investment*. A child who's healthy can go to school. A child who's healthy in school is more likely to do well. A child who does well in school is more likely to get a job. And people with jobs are less likely to end up in jail or on public assistance. *Thus, CHIP helps America to compete*. Ensuring that kids have health coverage is an investment in America's future.[45] (emphasis added)

And Senator Edward Kennedy includes both the human capital frame, also with school as the intervening activity, and the working families frame in his statement at a Senate hearing in July 2006. His use of the term "vulnerable" refers to both children and their families in an economic sense.

What we can say is that this has been enormously successful. It is a quality health care program. It is reaching the most *vulnerable*. It is reflected not only in giving the children a healthy start, it is helping children to read the blackboard so that they can *learn better*, it is making sure that they are healthier when they go to school so that they are going to have better attendance and they are going to have better results in terms of their own academic achievements and accomplishments. . . . Primarily, these are the children of workers. We know that it goes up to, depending on the States, with a family of three, $31,000, $32,000, $33,000. We are getting to individuals who are *working, working hard*, and just cannot afford those kind of premiums and are increasingly *vulnerable* in not having that coverage.[46] (emphasis added)

Once these word clusters were flagged and counted, they were then inspected to see if they were indeed part of a specific framing argument. These inspections determined that the words selected to signify the framing concepts of "morality," "working families," and "education/investment" did indeed identify these frames. For example, the terms "learning," "school," and "workforce" did mark the argument that funding children's health care will help children to function in school and thereby prepare them for employment. However, the terms "cost-effective" and "investment" were often used to generally describe what a public insurance program should be and did not necessarily mark the argument that investing in children in the present will save on future health-care costs.

Findings about the frames. Three findings resulted from this analysis of the framing of the expansion of SCHIP in congressional committee hearings held between 2006 and 2009. First, there is variation among hearings in the number and type of frames used. Second, as noted above, the terms "investment" and "cost-effective" did not always signify the future-oriented economic argument that long-term savings would be realized by providing preventive or primary health care for children. Third, the "morality" frame was used much less often than were the other frames.

The variation among the hearings is related to both the topic of the hearings and the types of witnesses speaking. The use of these frames was found to differ among hearings on SCHIP reauthorization because the subjects, purposes, and the testifying witnesses at these hearings varied greatly. For example, there were two hearings on the Bush administration's August 17 directive,[47] which was discussed in Chapter

4. The topics included the effect of the directive on enrollment policy in the states, whether the CMS regulations were legally issued, and what the congressional response could be. The focus of the hearings was not on the value of the SCHIP program and so *none* of the frames were used in these hearings.

In addition, I found that these frames were primarily used by two kinds of policy actors: members of Congress and representatives of organizations advocating for an expansion of SCHIP eligibility and benefits. The two hearings in which these frames were used most frequently were a hearing entitled *Covering the Uninsured Through the Eyes of a Child* (February 12 and 14, 2007) and a March 27, 2007, hearing *Insuring Bright Futures: Improving Access to Dental Care and Providing a Healthy Start for Children*. Both were conducted by the Health Subcommittee of the House Energy and Commerce Committee.

The February hearing was held at the beginning of the Health Subcommittee's consideration of the reauthorization of SCHIP and was one of the only hearings at which members of the committee made remarks. It is for these reasons that the numbers of these key words were the highest of any hearing, except the hearing on dental care. The term "working families" or "hard-working parents" was used eleven times in the hearing and twenty times in the prepared/written testimony. "School readiness," "learning," or "workforce" was mentioned thirteen times in the hearing and eleven times in the prepared testimony. The "investment frame" was used twenty-seven times in the hearing and thirty times in the written testimony.[48] In contrast, the vulnerable/moral frame—the words "vulnerable"/"vulnerability," "compassion"/"compassionate," and "moral"/"morality"—was only used five times in the hearing and four in the written testimony. (See Table 5.1.)

Table 5.1 Frames Used in *Covering the Uninsured Through the Eyes of a Child*, Congressional Hearing, February 12 and 14, 2007

Frame	Number of Times Cited in Hearing	Number of Times Cited in Testimony
Working families, hard-working parents	11	20
School readiness, learning, workforce	13	11
Investment	27	30
Vulnerable/moral	5	4

These same patterns were found in the hearing on including dental care in SCHIP. As discussed above, this hearing was held shortly after the death of Deamonte Driver, a twelve-year-old Maryland boy who died as a result of an infected tooth. His tragic death received a large amount of media coverage, and the imperative of preventing this type of tragedy again was discussed in the hearing. However, the hearing was also full of references to regular dental care as key to school performance. For example, Congresswoman Darlene Hooley, after discussing her shock and sadness at the death of Deamonte Driver, said,

> While we should shine a light on the heart wrenching tragedy of Deamonte's death, it is also important to remember that poor oral health has other consequences that are less severe but still detrimental to a child's well-being. As a former schoolteacher, I can attest to the fact that a child's toothache can have a very disruptive effect on the *learning process*. Not only is the child in pain, unable to learn, but a child in pain is often a disruptive force that hampers the ability of *other children to focus* and participate in class. That challenge to *effective learning* is unfortunately only part of the overall harm. In addition, more than 850,000 school days each year are missed by students because of dental-related illness. A child who is not in class obviously *cannot learn*. At a time when there is a strong emphasis on *student achievement*, I hope we can take an expansive view of what impacts *learning*. I think oral health is one of those factors that should get a lot more attention.[49] (emphasis added)

Even in the hearing held on oral health, the "morality-compassion" frame is only used eight times while the "school readiness/learning/workforce" set of key words is used thirty times. Interestingly, the term "working families" or "hard-working families" is not used at all during this hearing. The word "investment" was also used twenty-four times, sometimes in a very general sense (investment in health care) and sometimes as part of the argument that providing dental care is an investment in "human capital."

The testimonies given by five governors at a February 28, 2008, hearing of the House Committee on Energy and Commerce entitled *Covering Uninsured Kids: Reversing Progress Already Made* primarily focus on the issues of the SCHIP state funding formulas, the August 17 CMS letter to the states,[50] and other Bush administration policies and regulations related to the Medicaid program. Although little space was devoted to arguments about why a federal children's health insurance program should be reauthorized and/or expanded, the few general statements that were made about the value of SCHIP echoed the themes found in other hearings.

Deval L. Patrick, governor of Massachusetts, says, "quality healthcare enables children to better engage as students and fosters better lifelong health outcomes. These differences can set the course for a life."[51] Christine Gregoire, governor of Washington State, gave this testimony:

> I also came to understand not only the *moral* imperative of covering children, but the economic and societal benefits of doing so, as well. First, we learned that healthy children are *far* more likely to succeed in *school* and life—that the health of the next generation is critically important to the *future of our country*. . . . In Washington State, we believe that providing health care coverage to all of our kids and making sure they have access to high quality, affordable health care is not only the right thing to do—it is a *moral imperative*. We know that access to routine and preventive health care services can profoundly affect a child's health and well-being and *readiness for school. Healthy children learn better, grow better, and have a better chance of succeeding in life.*[52] (emphasis added)

Sonny Perdue, governor of Georgia, not only uses the "working families" frame, but also makes explicit the values that the frame represents: "SCHIP is not a government handout. It is not for unemployed families on welfare. It helps the children *of working parents* who not only pay their taxes, but who also pay premiums for the insurance their children receive."[53]

Very few of these frames were used when witnesses at a hearing were government administrators talking about technical issues. A Senate hearing on November 16, 2006, entitled *CHIP Program from the States' Perspective* focused on the issues of federal allocation of funds to the states, shortfalls in funding, and the specifics of the administration of the states' programs. Most of the witnesses discussing these topics were state Medicaid and SCHIP program administrators. There were only four references to "working families" and three to "vulnerable" children in the entire hearing and testimonies, and no framing at all in terms of school readiness/workforce investment.[54]

Similarly, in a House hearing on SCHIP on January 29, 2008, several months after the failure to override President Bush's 2007 vetoes, very few of these frames were used. The hearing focused on the history of children's coverage under SCHIP, the history of the 2007 legislative effort to reauthorize the program, and the effect that the August 17 CMS directive would have on children's coverage.[55] Five out of the seven witnesses were academic policy experts or state or federal government officials. The one representative from a national children's advocacy group, Bruce Lesley, the president of First Focus, framed the reauthorization of an expanded children's health insurance program as an "investment" in the future health of the US adult population:

> This is an American issue that affects not only our children but all of our futures. It is also a choice between investing now in improving the health and well-being of America's children or dealing with the effects of childhood obesity, growing levels of children's diabetes, and the lack of preventable disease when today's young people become adults. (Lesley 2008)

The morality frame. The finding that the morality frame was used much less often than the other frames can be explained in two ways. One is that the more "pragmatic" frames are viewed as more effective in attracting support for children's programs in 2007 as compared to the 1980s because of shifts in the political environment. This is the suggestion made by William T. Gormley Jr. in a paper reporting on his experimental study of responses to "economic" and "morality" frames used to attract support for a home visiting program (Gormley 2010) and in his 2012 book *Voices for Children*.[56] The reasons that he gives for such a change are growing concern about national budget deficits, the very large increase in the availability of policy data over time, ethnic heterogeneity, and the secularization of US society (Gormley 2012: ch. 2).

The other explanation, which is limited to this analysis, is that the method of looking for key words in the text can miss the morality frame because the appeal to compassion on behalf of vulnerable children may be made more effectively with the use of "stories" (Stone 2012). Thus, in the statement of the governor of Montana, quoted earlier, he conveyed a sense of children's vulnerability by saying "all over Montana there are young families who say a prayer with their children as they tuck them into bed, and after they tuck their children in, they go down the hall and they kneel again and they say a prayer." The vulnerability of children is conveyed without using that word and compassion is indeed evoked.

Similarly, the testimony of a thirteen-year-old, whose parents have a small business and who is one of five children, suggests vulnerability:

> I feel a little sad about having asthma because it limits the things I can do. I cannot play certain sports that require a lot of endurance. . . . But those are small worries compared to the ability to get health care. Having good health care through the Children's Health Insurance Pro-

gram means the health care that my siblings and I need is available to us. *There are no words to describe how safe that makes me feel.*[57] (emphasis added)

A pediatrician at the Children's Clinic in Billings, Montana, testifying at the same April 2007 Senate Finance Committee field hearing, used several powerful vignettes to present the dire personal and economic consequences of lack of regular medical care.

> What is life like for a child who does not receive medical care? Unfortunately, I have a lot of examples from my practice. One is the plight of a toddler with such rotten teeth and infected ears that he went on to develop mastoiditis, an exquisitely painful and life-threatening infection of the bone behind the ear. Or there is the teenage diabetic who shared her insulin with her uninsured diabetic family member to the detriment of them both. Another situation is one of an asthmatic teenager who made annual trips by airplane for about 3 years to a Billings hospital to spend a couple of days on life support before picking up a new supply of asthma medication, which he had depleted long ago. That is an expensive trip to the pharmacy. All of these cases have common elements. First, loving but economically challenged families were involved. Secondly, all cases represent common childhood maladies that were left unattended and became life-threatening. Third, the cost of these cases to our health care system and our State was staggering. And, finally, the single most important element in all these situations is that they could have been prevented by providing these children with regular access to routine medical surveillance and care.[58]

The vulnerability of children and compassion for them is an underlying, if unstated, theme.

In contrast to advocates of SCHIP expansion, who framed children's health insurance in terms of its benefits to children and to the economic future of the country, opponents placed the expansion of SCHIP within the larger context of debates about the boundaries of government health care.

Framing Opposition to SCHIP Expansion: Guarding the Border

As discussed in Chapter 3, SCHIP was created, in part, as an incremental response to the failure of the Clinton administration's attempt at health-care reform. Children's health insurance was on the agenda in

2007 because the 1997 SCHIP authorization was expiring, but it was also a period in which more extensive health-care reform was again on the agenda (Starr 2011). Congressional Democrats and advocacy groups wanted to use the reauthorization process to expand the program, and opposition to this expansion was framed in terms of the more general issue of "health reform" and the future structure of the health-care system. President Bush and some conservative members of Congress maintained that SCHIP should be limited to very low income children and viewed SCHIP expansion as a dangerous move toward "government medicine."

Framing Opposition and Health Reform

In remarks at the White House on September 20, 2007, President Bush said that he was opposed to the legislation that Congress had passed because it would cover children from higher-income families, was costly, and would increase government involvement in health care. "The compromise SCHIP plan is 'an incremental step toward the goal of government-run health care for every American,' the president said" (Teske 2007h). As described in the previous chapter, the president's two SCHIP veto messages used very similar language.

The congressional Republican leadership and officials of the Bush administration made this same argument: that expanding SCHIP would be crossing the border into the land of government medicine. Regional directors of the Department of Health and Human Services wrote letters to the editors about SCHIP expansion as a "government takeover of the health care marketplace" (quoted in Pear 2007). A July 2007 policy brief by the Senate Republican Policy Committee stated that the Democratic plan to increase the cigarette tax to pay for SCHIP reauthorization "is yet another in a growing list of examples where Democrats are working to expand federal entitlement programs to arrive, by the way of the back door, at government-run health care" (quoted in Teske 2007c). At an event sponsored by the Health Care Freedom Coalition, Congressman Mike Pence (R-IN) said the expansion of SCHIP would "condemn more children to government-run health care" and that 110 conservative members of Congress were engaging in a fight against it. Pence makes it clear that the opposition to SCHIP expansion is tied to the larger issue of health-care reform. "We are at the beginning of a national debate," he said. "Free market principles, or command and control principles?" (BNA 2007g). And in response to the passage of the first reauthorization bill in the House on August 1, 2007, secretary of the DHHS Michael O. Leavitt said that the bill would "move millions of children from private insurance *to public assistance* and create a *new middle-class entitlement* that our country cannot afford" (quoted in Teske and Hyland 2007, emphasis added).

Policy experts from the Heritage Foundation framed the expansion of SCHIP—even its existence—as steps toward a form of state-controlled medicine. SCHIP, they say, involves "'mission creep' toward national health insurance." And national health insurance, they argue, "would inevitably be characterized by central planning, price controls, rationing and the suppression of personal freedom." It is crossing the boundaries by expanding eligibility levels that is critical. States that have set income eligibility at or above 300 percent of the FPL "are turning middle-class families into welfare recipients at the expense of families in other states and taxpayers" (Marshner and Owcharenko 2007).

Framing Opposition and the Culture Wars

Although this was not a frame used by the Bush administration, it is very interesting to note that the same policy experts at the Heritage Foundation also used a "culture war" frame in arguing against the expansion of SCHIP. In the same WebMemo quoted earlier, they argue that "SCHIP has eroded a responsibility traditionally reserved to parents."

> Parents are the moral as well as the legal guardians of their children and have ultimate responsibility for their children's well-being. Yet, if children are enrolled in a government health program, the parents' options are set by government officials; these determinations are sometimes made on the basis of ideological or political calculations, not simply medical services. (Marshner and Owcharenko 2007)

The services that they are most concerned about are those related to "sexual behavior and health." This frame of governmental involvement as undermining parental responsibility and "traditional" family life is an echo of the Minority Chapter on Health Care of the 1991 Final Report on the National Commission on Children, discussed in Chapter 2.

In general, conservative opponents of the program were framing their opposition to expanding SCHIP in terms of the US ideological and political tradition that rigidly divides private and public medicine and limits public sector responsibility to those who are proven to have a low income through means tests. However, in earlier historical periods when opponents of expanding the government's role in providing health insurance or health services used this type of frame, they were doing so to protect their economic interests (see Marmor 2000; Quadagno 2005). This was not the case here.

Framing Opposition: Structural Interests and Ideology

First, there were apparently no organized economic or professional interest groups in the health field that opposed SCHIP expansion. On the contrary, in addition to the American Academy of Pediatrics and the National Association of Children's Hospitals, which advocated for the SCHIP expansion, the health insurance and pharmaceutical industries, the American Medical Association, as well as corporate groups such as the Business Roundtable were "on board" in support. As discussed earlier, PhRMA, the trade association for the major drug companies, paid for a large number of media advertisements calling for SCHIP reauthorization. And the representative of the trade group for Medicaid managed care companies visited congressional offices arm-in-arm with the representative of the AAP.

Laura Katz Olson's analysis of the "Medicaid medical industrial complex" can be applied to the trade associations that so wholeheartedly supported the efforts to expand SCHIP (Olson 2010: 181–184). Contrary to the perspective of the Bush administration, SCHIP subsidized the inclusion of more children into the private, profit-making health-care system and therefore created greater opportunities for payments to providers, including managed-care companies, hospitals, doctors, medical equipment companies, and pharmaceutical companies, among others. During earlier political struggles against the expansion of public health insurance coverage and/or health directly provided by public institutions, groups that believed that their economic interests were threatened used ideological opposition to "government medicine" to defend those interests. In contrast, in the case of SCHIP, health-care providers viewed expanded coverage as in their interest. The conservative opposition to SCHIP expansion seems to have been rooted in strictly ideological disagreement and linked to the larger, looming debate over health insurance reform.[59]

This opposition came from the Bush administration, conservative Republican members of Congress, and conservative think tanks. As noted in Chapter 3, this type of purely ideological opposition was mounted by conservative Republican intellectual leaders against the Clinton health-care plan, beginning in 1993. Rather than opposition to specific aspects of the plan, these Republican strategists attacked the concept of government expansion and lobbied the American Medical Association to oppose it, rather than vice versa (see Skocpol 1997).

While this ideological opposition in 2007 took place against a backdrop of the partisan ideological polarization that had begun decades earlier and was strategically fostered by Congressman Newt Gingrich in the 1980s and 1990s (Mann and Orenstein 2012), President Bush's two vetoes of the SCHIP reauthorization are in sharp contrast to his policy of expanding funding for the community health center (CHC) program. This was a federal grant program created during the War on Poverty by the Johnson administration and championed by Senator Edward Kennedy throughout his Senate career.

In 2001, in his first year in office, Bush proposed a five-year initiative to expand community health center sites to serve 6.1 million new patients, the largest of only two domestic public health programs that grew during the Bush administration (a much smaller program funded abstinence-only sex education). While the policy network supportive of the CHC program had included conservative members of Congress since the 1980s, two conservatives, Senator Christopher "Kit" Bond of Missouri (R) and Representative Henry Bonilla (R) of Texas had, in fact, tutored George W. Bush on the value of the health center model during his first campaign for the presidency, urging him to make it his signature health issue (Sardell 2012).

If his actions were based on a consistent desire to limit the government's role in health care, why would he initiate the expansion of the CHC program? The difference between Bush's actions on community health centers and SCHIP can be explained first in terms of the fact that conservative Republican allies convinced Bush that support for CHCs was a positive policy in the health arena. Second, community health centers provide access to medical care to individuals without health insurance and those in medically underserved areas (through both Medicaid and a federal categorical grant) *based on income level*. Thus, it can be argued that conservative Republicans can support this program because it actually reinforces the border between public and private medicine—or at the very least, doesn't challenge it. The expansion of SCHIP eligibility, on the other hand, threatens to violate that border.

The framing of SCHIP and Medicaid programs as "government medicine" by the Bush administration and some Republican members of Congress is quite ironic, given that about three-quarters of the children in SCHIP were receiving health services through a managed-care organization (Olson 2010: 299, footnote 118), the majority of which are owned by for-profit companies.

Framing in Editorials: Debate About the Boundaries

In addition to analyzing the way that SCHIP was framed by members of Congress, governors, academics, representatives of interest groups, and the Bush administration, I examined the words of another set of policy actors: editorial writers in regional and national newspapers. This was an effort to see which, if any, of the frames used by children's health advocates were accepted and used in editorials. Again I found that context was central: these writers accepted the value of children's health insurance and were responding to the president's veto and his arguments about the boundaries between public and private medicine.

The method used to analyze congressional hearings was used to analyze all editorials on SCHIP published in national and regional newspapers during that same period of time, 2007–2009. Surprisingly, the editorials written about the SCHIP reauthorization process did not frame the issue in the way that members of Congress did. Instead, in most cases, editorial writers *assumed the value of providing health insurance for children* and instead engaged directly in the ideological arguments about what part of the population should receive that coverage.

All of the editorials published between January 1, 2007, and February 28, 2009, in the twelve national and regional newspapers with the largest circulations[60] were reviewed and analyzed using the same coding scheme used to analyze congressional hearings. There were fifty-seven editorials written about the SCHIP reauthorization during this period.[61] Just under 50 percent of these editorials appeared in the *Washington Post* or the *New York Times*.

The terms that represent arguments about the unique qualities of children ("innocent," "vulnerable," "compassion") were rarely used. "Vulnerable" was used only twice, "compassion" twice, and "immoral" once. ("Preventing poor kids from seeing a doctor is deeply immoral.") The terms denoting the "deservedness" of children's parents ("working families" or "hard-working parents") were never used, nor were the terms that represent arguments about the long-term social gains that would result from providing health care to children: "school readiness," "learning," "competitiveness." Only three of the fifty-seven editorials make the kind of arguments for children's coverage that were made in advocating for Medicaid expansion during the 1980s and the creation of SCHIP in 1997. "The formula is quite simple: Healthier children make healthier adults. They do better in school. They fare better in life. Children with health care coverage also save on medical costs because they're not burdening emergency rooms with minor illnesses. Plus, those minor illnesses can be treated before they become major and costly." And parents "use Healthy Families to get their kids off to a good start in life and correct any problems that, left untreated, would turn into a larger taxpayer burden down the road" (*Los Angeles Times*, October 8, 2007).

Instead, almost all of the editorials responded to the ideological framing of the SCHIP program by the Bush administration and to the actions that the president and Republican members of Congress took in support of their position. The wisdom and moral rightness of providing health care for children does not appear as an explicit part of the discourse, but is implicitly claimed by both sides. The debate is rather about how this will be done without breaching the ideological boundaries between public and private medicine by raising SCHIP eligibility to cover the "middle class."

Most (88 percent) of the editorials were published during 2007, the year of the greatest congressional and administration activity on SCHIP reauthorization. More than half (56 percent, or thirty-two) discussed the ideological differences between the Bush administration and the majority of members of Congress on the expansion of SCHIP, and argued for or against the Bush vetoes. These editorials explicitly responded to President Bush's argument that the expansion of SCHIP would be a step toward universal, government-sponsored health care. Some supported the veto, others argued that although they did not support government-sponsored universal coverage, SCHIP expansion was far more limited and opposed the Bush veto. For example, the *Chicago Tribune* said on July 29, 2007,

> President Bush and Congress are on a collision course over something that most Americans would agree is a good thing: government-sponsored health insurance for poor children. The argument is not just about money—although that's a big part of it—but about overarching questions surrounding how far government should go to provide such coverage.

The *Arizona Republican* clearly rejects the Bush administration charge that SCHIP expansion is "socialized medicine," but nevertheless concludes that SCHIP should not be expanded to the "middle class."

> However, government programs to provide subsidized access to what is still a private system of health-care providers are very distinct from European-style national health-care systems. Moreover, federal tax policy also heavily subsidizes private, employer-provided health insurance. So, this is not a clean choice between public and private approaches. At the end of the rhetoric, however, congressional Democrats aren't proposing to reauthorize a program to insure low-income children. Instead, they are proposing a massive expansion of subsidized health care to middle-class families, funded by a large increase in heavily regressive tobacco taxes. That's an unwise, unfair and fiscally risky scheme.

Typical of those supporting the president's vetoes was the idea that only the "working poor" should be covered. An editorial in the *Dallas Morning News* on October 17, 2007, illustrates this point. "We supported the president's veto because the legislation would take the program beyond its original goal of helping working poor families cover their kids. We still think the focus needs to be on those children in families who earn $40,000 or less, which the program aimed to do when Congress passed it in 1997."

The opposite position is presented in an editorial in the *Houston Chronicle,* which urges members of the Texas congressional delegation, particularly from the Houston area, to vote for 2009 SCHIP legislation. This editorial does use the "cost-effective" and "investment" arguments as part of the rebuttal of the Bush ideological framing.

> In opposing SCHIP on the grounds it is socialized medicine, too costly and subsidizes illegal alien health care, the lawmakers are ignoring this fact: Taxpayers already bear the cost of treatment for the uninsured. Every child covered by the state-supplied private policies is one less expense for area health care providers, who otherwise pass the cost of indigent care on to insured patients. . . . Young Texans are the state's future workers, taxpayers and leaders. They need every opportunity to lead healthy, productive lives, and one of the surest guarantees that a child will successfully grow to adulthood is good medical care. In opposing SCHIP expansion, lawmakers are putting their ideology above the interests of their constituents.

The second largest category of editorial (ten in this category) also engaged in discussion of the Bush position and the arguments made by the administration, but were commenting on the August 17 directive. They were uniformly critical of this action. (Two editorials discussed both the veto and the August 17 directive.) The remainder of the editorials (seven) urged support for a particular House or Senate bill or for a provision of a bill, such as the inclusion of dental services within SCHIP.

Summarizing the Framing of SCHIP Expansion

Clearly, proponents and opponents of SCHIP expansion used very different types of frames in discussing the program. Advocates for the expansion of federally supported children's health insurance framed it in terms of the morality of caring for children, the cost-effectiveness of prevention and early treatment, and as an investment in school readiness and the future labor force. These were the same arguments used by advocates for the expansion of Medicaid eligibility and benefits for children in the mid and late 1980s and of the creation of SCHIP in 1997. Advocates for expansion were not framing their arguments in terms of broader health-care reform, but rather in terms of the specific characteristics of children and children's health services.

In stark contrast, the opponents of SCHIP expansion framed it as a "Trojan horse" of "government medicine," using the antigovernment rhetoric employed by opponents of expanding health-care coverage throughout the twentieth century. For the president and the Republican leadership in Congress, raising the income eligibility level for SCHIP beyond 200 percent or 250 percent of the FPL meant crossing an ideological boundary between private and public medicine. In the period 2007–2009, opponents of SCHIP expansion were viewing SCHIP as the first battle in the much larger fight about universal health-care reform.

Notes

1. See http://ccf.georgetown.edu/index/supporters.
2. See www.firstfocus.net.
3. Interview, First Focus staff, December 2, 2010.
4. Ibid.
5. Interview, AAP staff #4, November 11, 2010.
6. Ibid.
7. Ibid.; interview, Families USA staff #2, December 2, 2010.

8. Interview, AAP staff #4, November 11, 2010.
9. Interview, AAP staff #4, November 11, 2010; interview, First Focus staff, December 2, 2010.
10. Interview, AAP staff #4, November 11, 2010.
11. Ibid.
12. Ibid.
13. Interview, Families USA staff #2, December 2, 2010.
14. Ibid.
15. Ibid.
16. In 2009, PhRMA worked on the media campaign with the American Cancer Society and the Service Employees International Union (SEIU), as well as Families USA (interview, PhRMA policy staff, December 3, 2010). According to Robert Pear of the *New York Times,* the national trade associations of nursing homes and for-profit hospitals and the AMA joined with PhRMA and Families USA in spending on ads supportive of SCHIP expansion (Pear 2007).
17. Interview, PhRMA policy staff, December 3, 2010.
18. PhRMA Senate letter, January 31, 2007. In a similarly supportive letter to Congressman John Dingell, chair of the House Energy and Commerce Committee, on March 13, 2007, the emphasis was also on supporting provisions that provided funding for expanded state outreach and enrollment (PhRMA House letter, March 13, 2007).
19. Interview, PhRMA policy staff, December 3, 2010.
20. Interview, Families USA staff #2, December 2, 2010.
21. Ibid.
22. Interview, AAP staff #4, November 11, 2010.
23. Interview, Senate Republican staff #6, December 2, 2010.
24. Ibid.
25. Interview, Families USA staff #2, December 2, 2010.
26. Interview, First Focus staff, December 2, 2010.
27. Interview, AAP staff #4, November 11, 2010.
28. Ibid.
29. CCF (2009).
30. In 2013 Edelstein was professor of dentistry in the College of Dental Medicine and Health Policy and Management in the Mailman School of Public Health at Columbia University.
31. See Govtrack.us.
32. Interview, AAP staff #4, November 11, 2010.
33. See Gormley 2012 (pp. 131–133) for a discussion of Deamonte's death as an example of a "compelling story" and differing policy responses to it by Democratic and Republican staffers that he interviewed. I found similar differences by political party during my interviews with congressional staff.
34. See Govtrack.us.
35. The only opposition to a federally mandated oral health provision came from the National Governors Association and Republican House members who objected to more federal requirements put on the states.

36. While Democrats had a clear majority in the House, the Senate was split forty-nine Democrats to forty-nine Republicans, with two independents who voted with the Democrats.

37. All of the hearings on SCHIP that were available electronically during July 2009 were downloaded from the Senate and House committee websites. These included six House hearings in 2007 and 2008 and seven Senate hearings from 2006 through 2009.

38. This was done because the actual hearings included shorter, more informal testimony from the witnesses as well as short opening presentations from subcommittee/committee members and exchanges between the members of Congress and the witnesses. Informal statements made in the presence of members of Congress within a real-time context may differ somewhat from the written testimony.

39. *Children's Health Insurance Program in Action: A State's Perspective on CHIP: Hearing Before the S. Comm. on Fin.*, 110th Cong. (April 4, 2007).

40. Gormley analyzed Edelman's congressional testimony over a forty-year period and found both "moralistic" and "economic" arguments (Gormley 2012: 31–33).

41. *Children's Health Insurance Program in Action: A State's Perspective on CHIP: Hearing Before the S. Comm. on Fin.*, 110th Cong. (April 4, 2007).

42. Ibid.

43. Both the human capital and cost-effective frames were used by advocates arguing in 2003 for a reversal of the five-year ban on legal immigrant children and pregnant women: pregnant women without prenatal care are far more likely to have low–birth weight and premature babies; uninsured pregnant women and children are more likely to be hospitalized for conditions that can be managed without hospitalization and thus are more costly for the health-care system; and children with health coverage are more likely to be treated for conditions that interfere with learning and thus to do better in school and have greater "economic and social success" than uninsured children (Families USA 2003b).

44. *The Future of CHIP: Improving the Health of America's Children: Hearing Before the S. Comm. on Fin.*, 110th Cong. (February 1, 2007).

45. *Open Executive Session to Consider the CHIP Reauthorization Act of 2007: Hearing Before S. Comm. on Fin.*, 110th Cong. (July 19, 2007). For the Senate Finance Executive Session hearing on July 19, 2010, the only parts of the hearing that are available electronically are the statements of the chair and ranking member of the committee. The working families frame was used three times, the competitive/school readiness frame four times.

46. *CHIP at 10: A Decade of Covering Children*: *Hearing Before the Subcomm. on Health Care of the S. Comm. on Finance*, 109th Cong. (July 25, 2006).

47. *HR 5998 Protecting Children's Health Coverage of 2008: Hearing Before the Subcomm. on Health of the H. Comm. on Energy and Commerce*, 110th Cong. (May 15, 2008); *Covering Uninsured Children: The Impact of the August 17 CHIP Directive: Hearing Before the Subcomm. on Health of the S. Comm. on Fin.*, 110th Cong. (April 9, 2008).

48. The words "cost-effective" were used nine times in the hearing and eleven times in the written testimony, and the word "investment" was used fourteen times during the hearing and nineteen times in the prepared testimony, but as noted earlier, sometimes the word "investment" was not specifically used as an argument for children's health insurance.

49. *Insuring Bright Futures: Improving Access to Dental Care and Providing a Healthy Start for Children: Hearing Before the Subcomm. on Health of the H. Comm. on Energy and Commerce,* 110th Cong. (March 27, 2007).

50. Three of the governors asked members of Congress to rescind or nullify the August 17 directive, and one governor, Haley Barbour of Mississippi, supported it.

51. *Covering Uninsured Kids: Reversing Progress Already Made: Hearing Before the H. Comm. on Energy and Commerce*, 110th Cong. (February 26 and 28, 2008).

52. Ibid.

53. Ibid.

54. *CHIP Program from the States' Perspective: Hearing Before the Subcomm. on Health Care of the S. Comm. on Fin.,* 109th Cong. (November 16, 2006).

55. *Covering Uninsured Kids: Missed Opportunities for Moving Forward: Hearing Before the Subcomm. on Health of the H. Comm. on Energy and Commerce,* 110th Cong. (January 29, 2008).

56. Gormley finds two distinct "moralistic" arguments: the "helping-hand" and the "equal opportunity" arguments.

57. *Children's Health Insurance Program in Action: A State's Perspective on CHIP: Hearing Before the S. Comm. on Fin.,* 110th Cong. (April 4, 2007).

58. Ibid.

59. Jonathan B. Oberlander and Barbara Lyons use the term "boundary issues" to describe the ideological divide over SCHIP expansion in a 2009 article and warn that this may reoccur in the upcoming debate over universal health reform (Oberlander and Lyons 2009).

60. The list was based on daily circulation for the six months ending March 2010. The newspapers included are the *New York Times, Los Angeles Times,* the *Washington Post, San Jose Mercury News, Chicago Tribune, Houston Chronicle, Arizona Republic, Philadelphia Inquirer, Denver Post, Star Tribune, St. Petersburg Times,* and *Dallas Morning News.* Only one paper was selected from the same city. Thus, the *Wall Street Journal, USA Today, Daily News, New York Post,* and the *Philadelphia Daily News* were not included in the list even though their circulations are higher than some of the newspapers that were included. I want to express my gratitude to Gerald Solomon, professor in the Journalism Program of Queens College, CUNY, for his help in selecting this list.

61. Editorials that focused solely on state-level policy decisions about children's health insurance were excluded from this analysis; editorials that discussed state data and programs in the context of the federal policy process on reauthorization were included.

6

The State of Children's Health

In this book, I recount the history of the activities, the debates, and the decisions that resulted in an increasing expansion of public health-insurance coverage for children in the United States during the past three decades. Although Americans support health care for children more than for any other group,[1] this history is filled with ideological and partisan conflict about the boundaries of the public and private health-care sectors and the power of states versus the federal government. It is also a policy history that illustrates the critical importance of policy entrepreneurs—both inside and outside government—in identifying and framing problems, proposing policy solutions for those problems, and responding to shifts in the larger political environment. The longitudinal perspective of this project has enabled me to trace the ways in which policy conflicts and decisions at one point in time became policy legacies in the form of social learning at later points. This study clearly shows the key roles of both "substantive" and "situational" social learning in the policymaking process, as well as the importance of framing as an advocacy strategy on behalf of a "resourceless" group such as low-income children.

During the 1980s, policy entrepreneurs such as Marian Wright Edelman, Governor Richard W. Riley of South Carolina, Congressman George E. Miller, and Senator Lawton Chiles created or led institutions whose work focused attention on the services needed to assure that children were healthy and on policy arguments about why that was important to America's future. Public institutions such as the National Commission to Prevent Infant Mortality and private groups such as the Children's Defense Fund and the Ford Foundation framed the need to provide access to health care for pregnant women and children in terms of the moral imperative to reduce infant mortality, the "cost-effectiveness" of services that would prevent childhood disability, and the importance of investment in children as future members of the US workforce. These frames were policy legacies, the substantive learning about children's health that was the basis for the creation of the State Children's Health Insurance Program (SCHIP) in 1997 and its reauthorization as the Children's Health Insurance Program in 2009. Advocates for SCHIP expansion in 2007 used similar frames, although the frequency of the use of specific frames varied over time.

"Situational" learning occurs as prior events influence the views of policy actors about the political consequences of their actions. The victory of Republicans in the 1994 election and the subsequent nearly successful transformation of the Medicaid program from an entitlement to a block grant operated as situational policy legacies for the Children's Defense Fund and Senator Edward Kennedy, the policy entrepreneurs driving forward a children's health insurance program that was not a federal entitlement. In addition to the formulation of this proposal and the creation of a committed legislative partnership between a liberal Democrat, Senator Edward Kennedy, and a conservative Republican, Senator Orrin Hatch, the third part of the entrepreneurial strategy for the advancement of the children's health-insurance proposal was its framing. The targets of the program were socially constructed as the children of "hard-working parents" and it was linked to the campaign conducted by public health groups against the encouragement of youthful smoking by cigarette companies.

I have also examined changes within the child health advocacy coalition over time. There was a shift in the leadership of the inner core of the coalition, the creation of both a new children's bipartisan advocacy group and a new think tank, and several broader coalitions formed to work for SCHIP expansion during the 2007–2009 reauthorization process. That process also shows how policy communities concerned about particular issues (access to dental care, coverage for legal immigrant pregnant women and children, and quality measures for pediatric care) used the reauthorization as a "window of opportunity" as discussed by John Kingdon (1995).

In addition, the case of children's health insurance illustrates how policy is a result of the interaction of policy communities with the broader political environment, or "political stream." The 1996 midterm elections that resulted in continued conservative Republican control of Congress in 1997 limited the possibility of the expansion of health insurance for low-income children through a federal entitlement. Similarly, the expansion of the federal children's health insurance program was not possible until the election of 2008 brought a Democratic president to the White House and more Democrats to Congress.

Children's health insurance was not an isolated issue but was related to efforts to achieve universal coverage. When the "health reform" efforts of Democratic presidents failed, children's advocates, federal officials, and members of Congress viewed covering children as the next step in an incremental strategy toward universal health insurance. In the late 1970s, an expansion of Medicaid eligibility for pregnant women and children was proposed by children's advocates inside and outside of the Carter administration when it was clear that a broader expansion of public health coverage would not be enacted. The same dynamic occurred when Congress created SCHIP in 1997 after the failure of the Clinton administration's health plan. The contentiousness and stalemate over SCHIP reauthorization in 2007 was related to the broader debate over the structure of US health care that was emerging, as well as the partisan and ideological polarization that had been increasing since the 1990s.

That ideological polarization is seen in President George W. Bush's two vetoes of SCHIP reauthorization bills in 2007, in the August 17 administrative directive issued by his administration, and in the antigovernment frames used to explain opposition to SCHIP expansion. This was the same antigovernment rhetoric that opponents of health-care reform had used at several past junctures in the history of US health policy. In 2007, this framing was employed against anticipated, rather than actual, structural change. And in contrast to prior framing of legislation proposing universal health insurance as "anti-American, socialized medicine" by structural interests in the health-care industry, physicians, insurance companies, and the pharmaceutical industry were all active supporters of the expansion of children's health insurance.

It is interesting to now briefly comment on the question of whether the creation and expansion of SCHIP are a case of policy change or policy continuity in the terms discussed by Frank Baumgartner and Bryan Jones. Baumgartner and Jones (1993) developed a "punctuated equilibrium model of policy change" that explains how periods of stability within a specific policy arena can be interspersed with major policy shifts. Related policy actors who share a set of policy ideas constitute a "policy monopoly," which dominates a given policy domain but may later be replaced by a different set of policy ideas and a different set of policy actors or relationships. Baumgartner and Jones discuss several cases to illustrate their model, including the cases of nuclear power, pesticides, and smoking, all cases in which public beliefs about a product and an industry changed dramatically in response to alternative ideas within that policy area.

In some ways, the enactment of SCHIP can be seen as marking a new era in US child health policy. The Balanced Budget and Revenue Reconciliation Acts of 1997 did allocate the largest amount of federal money to children's health since the passage of Medicaid three decades earlier. In fact, it was the biggest expansion of any federally financed health insurance since 1965 (McDonough 2011). SCHIP was (primarily) a children-only program, unlike Medicaid, which allots three-quarters of its expenditures to the care of elderly and disabled adults. To the extent that the creation of a separate federal child health program signaled the idea that children as a category should have health insurance coverage, the definition of the public health insurance universe was broadened. Children, like adults over age sixty-five, were to be included as groups that policy actors outside the children's health policy network agreed should be provided with health insurance.

But the enactment of SCHIP did not involve broad public involvement or the replacement of one set of policy ideas about child health with a different set of ideas. In fact, the theme of "insuring children" is just the opposite. The data presented in Chapters 2, 3, and 5 illustrate social learning by policy actors about the relationship of access to health services and child health status and the continuity of the framing over time. More significantly, the enactment and expansion of the SCHIP program *extended* the categorical structure of health insurance in the United States, as well as the tradition of using public money to buttress the existing private health-care system.

It is now time to very briefly reflect on the achievements and limitations of SCHIP and the Children's Health Insurance Program (CHIP) in expanding access to health care for children, as well as how children's health insurance coverage will be affected by the implementation of the Patient Protection and Affordable Care Act of 2010. Then it is important to step back and look at the broader issue of the state of children's health in the United States today. A comparison with other wealthy, postindustrial nations is enlightening, because we see that we rank last on many measures of health status, for both children and adults. A recent comparative analysis of health status in the United

States with seventeen other wealthy nations by the National Research Council and the National Institute of Medicine suggests that differences in the health system, the physical and social environment, the political culture, and even political structures contribute to the poorer state of children's health in the United States as compared to those other countries.

The Achievements and Challenges of SCHIP/CHIP

The major achievements of the State Children's Health Insurance Program (SCHIP) and the Children's Health Insurance Program Reauthorization Act (CHIPRA) have been the increased insurance coverage of children, including the enrollment of Medicaid-eligible children who were previously not enrolled. The increase in public coverage of children since 2000 is clearly seen in Figure 6.1.[2]

At the same time as the enactment of SCHIP and related efforts to enroll more children in both Medicaid and SCHIP increased children's coverage, the proportion of adults with health insurance has decreased. The major recession that began in December 2007 brought with it a loss of employer-based health insurance coverage to workers and their fam-

Figure 6.1 Children (under age 18) with Public Health Plan Coverage, 2000–2011

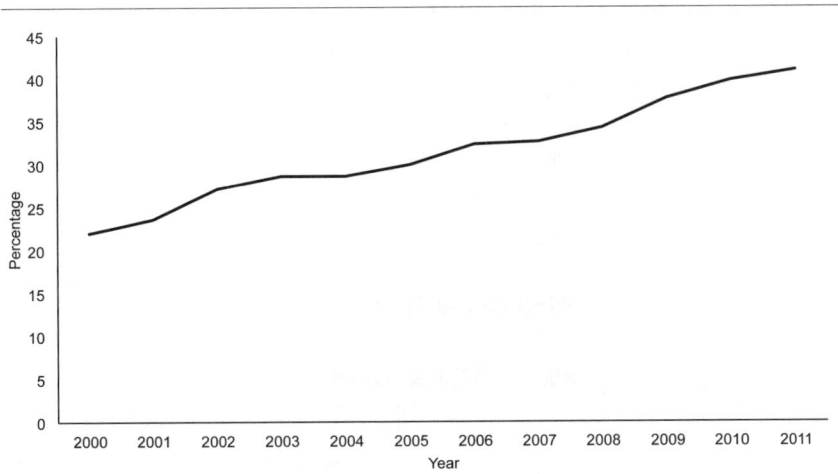

ilies, but Medicaid and SCHIP/CHIP continued to expand coverage for children. Between 2008 and 2011, the proportion of uninsured children decreased, even as the poverty rate for children increased (CCF 2012). Recent data from the National Health Interview Survey show the large differences in health insurance coverage for children as compared to adults. Adults were more than three times as likely as children to be uninsured at the time of the interview, more than twice as likely as children to be uninsured for at least part of the year, and more than four times as likely to be uninsured for more than a year (see Figure 6.2).

While the expansion of public insurance for children has protected many of them from the loss of coverage suffered by adults during the nation's long recession and continuing retrenchments in worker benefits, there are still large numbers of US children who remain uninsured. As of July 2012, 8 million children did not have health insurance. Five million of these children were eligible for Medicaid or CHIP but not enrolled (Kaiser Family Foundation 2012). Enrolling eligible children has been a long-term implementation challenge for both Medicaid and SCHIP. The 1997 SCHIP legislation provided funding to the states for outreach and enrollment activities, and as noted in Chapter 4, there was an unprecedented effort by the Clinton administration, foundations, and

Figure 6.2 Child and Adult Health-Insurance Coverage, January–September 2012

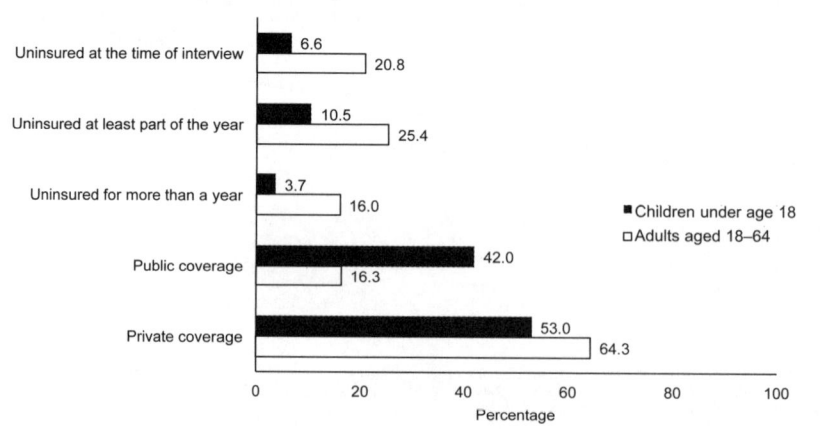

advocacy groups to encourage the states to use best practices in their enrollment efforts. States developed application forms and enrollment processes for SCHIP that were far simpler than the Medicaid application process and, in many states, simplified the Medicaid application process as well. There were enrollment efforts using local community-based organizations as well as mass media information campaigns. The result was a large increase in SCHIP enrollment from 1 million in 1998 to 5.3 million in fiscal year 2002. There was also an increase in Medicaid enrollment linked to the requirement that all children eligible for Medicaid must be enrolled in that program, even when their families applied to a separate state program.

However, it was not clear that the enrollment numbers reflected continuous enrollment and continuous access to care. Studies of retention in the early years of the program found that administratively complicated recertification procedures in some states resulted in disenrollment of as many as 50 percent of those enrolled at any one point in time (Ryan 2003). Efforts have been made since program reauthorization to reduce the considerable variation in the rate of enrollment of eligible children across the states. By the end of 2011, CHIPRA had provided $90 million in grants to provider groups, states, and community-based organizations for activities to increase enrollment and retention (CCF 2012).

Barriers to enrolling children in SCHIP/CHIP and Medicaid include the structure of federalism, negative attitudes about public benefits, and the related fears and attitudes of parents about enrollment. "Marketing challenges" include the historical failure of all levels of government to educate potential recipients about their eligibility for Medicaid and parental fear about legal status, concern about stigma, and the belief that they can access care without health insurance. In addition, states can be concerned that easing the enrollment process will result in the enrollment of children who are not, in fact, eligible, and this can result in opposition to such programs. There is also the fragmented nature of the process; in many states, local governments or several state departments are responsible for enrollment and may not all have the same commitment to enrollment expansion as do the federal or state governments (Thompson 2012: ch. 3).

In addition to expanding health-insurance coverage, SCHIP/CHIP has improved access to care. Embry Howell and Genevieve Kenney (2012) did a comprehensive review and synthesis of all of the quantitative peer-reviewed literature on the effects of the Medicaid expansions and SCHIP/CHIP, excluding studies that were not methodologically sound or did not estimate the size of these effects.³ Their analysis of the remaining thirty-eight studies concluded that in addition to the decline in the number of uninsured children, found in all studies, there was also a significant improvement in having a usual source of care for children who were enrolled in these programs.

However, solid data on whether and how SCHIP/CHIP has affected the quality of care and *the health status* of children are quite limited. The impact of these programs on health status is difficult to measure, in part because the effects of health care on children may not appear for many years. While the fewest number of studies were concerned with health status, there was also less evidence that Medicaid and SCHIP/CHIP affect health status than that they improve access to care. The studies that showed a positive impact of Medicaid/SCHIP on health status were limited to those that looked at child mortality and hospitalization. No studies were available of the way that different state delivery systems, provider payment, or cost-sharing affected children's health status. The *characteristics of health-care delivery systems* that positively affect health status are, of course, a critical policy issue. Another central issue, briefly discussed below, is that children's health status is a product of many economic, social, and environmental factors that are not necessarily wholly mitigated by access to health-care services.

As discussed previously, the American Academy of Pediatrics (AAP), National Association of Children's Hospitals and Related Institutions (NACHRI), and other policy actors advocated for the development of child health quality measures by the Department of Health and Human Services (DHHS). One of the provisions of CHIPRA was that a study be conducted by the Institute of Medicine and the National Research Council on the extent and quality of research on child health status and the quality of children's health care. Such a report done by the Committee on Pediatric Health and Health Quality Measures found that while there are many federal data sets, there is no "robust national information system that can provide timely, comprehensive, and valid and reliable indicators of health and health care quality for children and adolescents" (Institute of Medicine and the National Research Council 2011: 1). The report recommends to the secretary of DHHS that new measures be developed to assess relationships between social determinants of health and health status and the quality of health care, and that interagency cooperation be used to develop the capacity to use existing data sources to capture these relationships.

Going Forward:
The ACA and Children's Health Coverage

In addition to making the reauthorization of SCHIP possible, the 2008 election shifted the political stream so that the enactment of a national expansion of health-insurance coverage for both children and adults was accomplished in 2010. The Patient Protection and Affordable Care Act (ACA), PL 111-148, expands health-insurance coverage in several different ways. First, the ACA expands Medicaid eligibility for individuals and families with income up to 133 percent of the federal poverty level (which is actually 138 percent of the FPL based on the modified adjusted gross income) for all of those who are not eligible for Medicare. The federal government will pay for the full cost of this expansion from 2014 to 2016, a slightly decreasing amount through 2019, and then 90 percent of the cost for the newly eligible in 2020 and subsequently. The ACA also requires the states to create health-insurance exchanges through which individuals or families with incomes between 135 percent and 400 percent of the FPL can purchase coverage with subsidized tax credits (Kaiser Family Foundation 2013).

During the process of drafting the ACA,[4] there was debate over the future of CHIP. The question was whether CHIP should continue as a separate children's program or whether children, along with their families, should get coverage through the state insurance exchanges. The House bill would have repealed CHIP in 2014. Higher-income families (those with incomes over 150 percent of the FPL) would work with the exchanges and subsidies, and lower-income parents and their children (those with incomes less than 150 percent of the FPL) would be eligible for the expanded Medicaid program. Senator Max Baucus introduced a similar idea in the Finance Committee, with the addition that CHIP benefits that were not provided by health insurance companies within the exchanges would be provided by the states. The Senate champion of preserving CHIP as a separate program was Senator Jay Rockefeller, whose proposal to continue SCHIP and *increase* the federal matching rates to the states was incorporated into the majority leader's amendment and was enacted as part of the ACA (McDonough 2011). The result was that the ACA extends funding for the program through 2015 and requires that the states maintain current eligibility and benefit levels through 2019. Beginning in 2015, there will be a 23 percent increase in the CHIP match rate to the states, up to 100 percent (Kaiser Family Foundation 2013).

Other provisions of the ACA affect children who are already covered by private health insurance. As of September 23, 2010, all insurance companies are required to provide dependent coverage for adult children until age twenty-six, and the denial of coverage to a child based on a preexisting condition is prohibited. Beginning in 2014, insurers cannot establish lifetime coverage limits, so that ill children will not be barred from coverage when they are older. The ACA also requires that over time, children covered by private insurance receive preventive services. All private insurance plans established after September 2010 are required to cover a series of preventive services as defined by AAP standards, such as comprehensive screenings, preventive care, well-child care, and immunizations, all without any copayments. While existing plans are exempt from these standards, more children will be provided with comprehensive preventive services going forward. In addition, the ACA provides that children whose parents do not have children's coverage as part of their employer-provided coverage (or who live with their grandparents) can access individual children's coverage through the new health exchanges if they do not qualify for Medicaid or CHIP (First Focus 2013).

The question of the future impact of the ACA on children's coverage was the subject of a joint study by researchers at the Urban Institute and the Center for Children and Families at Georgetown University (Kenney et al. 2011). Using data from the 2009 and 2010 Current Population Survey, they used a microsimulation to estimate the effect of the implementation of the Affordable Care Act on different groups of children in the United States. The model predicted that increases in the number of children enrolled in Medicaid and CHIP and additional family coverage through the new state insurance exchanges (plus a small increase in employer-sponsored coverage) would result in a decline in the number of uninsured children from 7.5 million to 4.2 million, or from 9.4 to 5.3 percent of all children.[5] The largest declines in uninsured status would be for children in families with incomes of 138–250 percent of the FPL and Hispanic children. The decline would come from the enrollment in Medicaid and CHIP of children who were previously eligible but not enrolled, and from family coverage stimulated by the individual mandate and the establishment of state insurance exchanges. Almost half of all children would receive coverage through employer-sponsored insurance, 41 percent through Medicaid and CHIP, and 5 percent through exchange coverage. Of the approximately 5 percent of children who would still be uninsured, half would be eligible for Medicaid or CHIP but not enrolled, 15 percent would be undocumented immigrants, and one-third would be in families eligible for exchange coverage or employer-based coverage but not enrolled.

The expansion of Medicaid eligibility and, to a lesser extent, subsidized coverage through the state insurance exchanges would also reduce the number of uninsured parents by about half, from 12.7 million to 6.6 million. Children benefit when their parents have access to medical and mental-health care. Thus, these provisions of the ACA were in some ways a response to the debate over parental coverage under SCHIP and the opposition to it by Republican members of Congress.

This simulation, however, is based on continuation of the CHIP provisions of the ACA. The authors of this study also estimated the effect on children's health-insurance coverage if Congress does not continue to fund CHIP after fiscal year 2015. In that case, it is assumed that the states would dismantle their separate CHIP programs and this would mean the loss of coverage for 1.8 million to 2.4 million children. If the "maintenance of effort" requirement is rescinded, the estimate is that 7.9 million to 9.1 million children would be uninsured, *numbers greater than if the ACA had not been enacted.* In addition, those children whose families would be eligible for the exchanges or those covered by employer plans would probably have a poorer benefit plan and higher out-of-pocket costs than those receiving coverage through a public plan (Kenney et al. 2011).

The extreme polarization of Congress, and the US political system generally, continues and there is controversy over the implementation of the provisions of the ACA. In June 2012, the Supreme Court decided that the Medicaid expansion provisions of the ACA were constitutional, but it did not allow the federal government to require states to expand Medicaid. Thus, the states will determine whether adults with incomes up to 138 percent of the FPL will be covered, a decision that will affect many of the parents of children enrolled in Medicaid and CHIP. As of October 22, 2013, twenty-five states and the District of Columbia were enacting the Medicaid expansions, twenty-five were not (Kaiser Family Foundation 2013). However, the ACA requires that even if states do not expand Medicaid eligibility, they must put in place new enrollment processes. These processes will vastly simplify application and renewal—for example, by the use of a single national application that can be submitted online, electronic data matches to verify eligibility, and coordination with state insurance exchanges. These methods are meant to increase the numbers of eligible children receiving health insurance through Medicaid and CHIP.

Most significant for children is the ACA requirement, affirmed by the Supreme Court, that beginning in 2014, states are prohibited from reducing benefits or eligibility, or introducing cost-sharing for Medicaid and CHIP through 2019. This is the "maintenance of effort" provision (Kaiser Family Foundation 2013). This policy is one that congressional Republicans have attempted to reverse. Two Republican bills that reduced domestic spending passed the House in May 2012 and in December 2012. Both repealed ACA provisions prohibiting states from reducing eligibility levels for children covered by CHIP and Medicaid and provisions providing bonus payments to states for enrollment and retention activities for those two programs.[6] They were not, however, acted upon in the Senate, where Democrats had a majority.

Stepping back from this story of the efforts to expand children's health insurance coverage during the past three decades, I will briefly examine the existing state of the health of US children. I will then report on the comparative health status of children in other wealthy nations. This is a perspective that has been largely missing from the political debate over children's health services since the 1980s.[7]

US Children's Health Status: A Portrait of Disparities

Children under age eighteen constituted almost a quarter of the US population (23.7 percent) in 2011. A little over half (53.2 percent) were "white," 14 percent were "black," 4.4 percent were Asian, and almost a quarter (23.6 percent) were Hispanic. Looking at family situations, 65 percent were living with two married parents, while 23 percent were living with at least one foreign-born parent. Data from 2010 showed that 22 percent of children lived in households that were "food insecure," and 45 percent in families that indicated problems with housing or housing costs. In terms of money coming into the household, 22 percent of children under age eighteen and 25 percent of children under age six lived in families with incomes below the federal poverty level, which for a family of three was $18,310 in 2010. This was true for 39 percent of black children, 35 percent of Hispanic children, and 12 percent of white children (Federal Interagency Forum on Child and Family Health 2012).

The infant mortality rate in the United States in 2009 was 6.4 deaths per 1,000 live births. The rate among infants born to black women (including Hispanic women identifying themselves as black) was 12.71, almost two and a half times the rate for babies born to Hispanic women (5.3) and white women (5.4). Babies born at low birth weights are more likely to die in their first year of life and to have physical and developmental problems than babies born at normal weight. The rate of low birth weight in the United States in 2009 was 8.2. Again there were ethnic differences. The rate was much higher for infants of black women than for infants of women of any other ethnic group. This was also true for the rate of babies born at very low birth weight (less than 3 pounds 4 ounces). Such infants are 100 times more likely to die before their first birthday than are babies born at normal weight.

Chronic physical and mental health conditions in children, including learning disabilities, also vary by race and ethnicity. According to parental reports, 30 percent of non-Hispanic black children had one or more chronic conditions compared to 22.5 percent of non-Hispanic white children and 18.3 percent of Hispanic children. Parents of black children reported more severe asthma in their children than the parents of white children. Obesity among US children is a major public health concern: its prevalence increased threefold for girls and fourfold for boys during the past thirty years. Childhood obesity increases the risk for cardiovascular disease and Type 2 diabetes in children and for obesity in adulthood. Obesity in children varies by household income. In 2007, more than a quarter (27.4 percent) of children living in households with incomes below the federal poverty level were obese, compared to 10 percent of children living in households with incomes of 400 percent of the FPL or higher.

There are also inequalities in health-care coverage by social class and ethnicity. In 2009, 7.5 million children under eighteen, or about 10 percent of US children, had no health insurance. More than a third (36.8 percent) of children who were insured were covered by Medicaid and CHIP. Both being insured and being insured privately varied by family income and ethnicity. Hispanic children were the least likely to be insured. Having less than adequate coverage (as in a limited private plan) and having periods of noninsurance in a year also varied by income and age. Younger children were more likely to have adequate coverage.

Visits to health-care professionals also varied by income and ethnicity, for both medical and dental care. In 2009, almost 80 percent of children ages two through seventeen saw a dental provider, but 15 percent of children had not received *any dental care* in more than two years. A little more than 13 percent of children living in households with incomes below the poverty level had not seen a medical provider in the past year, compared to 5.4 percent of children living in households with income of 400 percent of the FPL or higher (DHHS 2012).

Not surprisingly, the "quality" of children's health care also appears to vary by family income. The AAP defines a "medical home" for children as health care that is "accessible, continuous, comprehensive, family centered, coordinated, compassionate and culturally effective" (DHHS 2012: 65). The National Survey of Children's Health in 2007 included questions to measure these qualities and found that almost 40 percent of children living in families with incomes less than the federal poverty level had a "medical home," compared to almost 70 percent of children in homes where the household income was at or above 400 percent of the FPL (DHHS 2012: 65).

Although access to high-quality health care improves health status, especially for populations with chronic disease or lower socioeconomic status (DHHS 2012: 65), there is now recognition that health-care disparities are embedded in broader structural inequalities that cannot be mitigated solely by improving access to health services. Disparities in health status are understood as occurring across the "life course" as early as preconception. Individual health behavior and exposure to health risks in the social and physical environment exist within the context of social and economic inequality in education, housing, land use, transportation, and the labor market (Rowley et al. 2013). These disparities are reflected in international data that place the United States at the bottom of the rankings for rates of infant mortality among wealthy, postindustrial nations.[8]

The Comparative Perspective

Although the United States spends far more than do most other countries on health-care services, Americans are relatively "disadvantaged" in health outcomes when compared to those of other high-income nations. For all ages up to seventy-five, US residents have shorter life expectancies than the residents of sixteen comparable countries—thirteen in Europe, plus Australia, Canada, and Japan (Woolf and Aron 2013). In a study entitled *U.S. Health in International Perspective: Shorter Lives, Poorer Health*, an interdisciplinary scientific panel convened by the National Research Council and Institute of Medicine reports on these differences and the broad environmental, social, and political factors that influence them. The lower life expectancy of residents of the United States is explained by an infant mortality rate that is the highest of all seventeen countries; death rates of children, adolescents, and young adults from homicide, traffic, and other accidents at higher rates than in other nations; higher rates of adolescent pregnancies, sexually transmitted diseases (including AIDS), and alcohol- and drug-related mortality; and higher rates of obesity, diabetes, heart disease, and chronic lung disease. Although this "health disadvantage" is greater for lower-income groups and ethnic minorities in the United States, highly educated, upper-income white Americans also have worse health than similar groups in the other nations.

The report discusses the "alarming scale of health disadvantage among children and adolescents in the United States compared with their peers in other high income countries" (Woolf and Aron 2013: 232). The pattern for many years has been that both infant mortality[9] and mortality after age fifteen are higher in the United States than in other comparatively wealthy countries. On a 2007 United Nations Children's Fund (UNICEF) score based on low birth weight, infant mortality, breastfeeding, physical activity, immunization, and youth suicide, the United States ranked twenty-one out of twenty-one countries. The US rate of adolescent pregnancy (which is related to low birth weight and infant mortality) in 2010 was almost 3.5 times the average rate in other wealthy nations; the probability of dying before age five is the highest of seventeen high-income countries.

The panel's report discusses several types of variables that explain this US health disadvantage when compared to other wealthy countries: the health-care system, lifestyle and individual behavior, the physical and social environment, and public policies. Their study suggests many ways in which these variables interact with one another. For instance, children living in poverty may have less access to preventive health care but more exposure to pollutants in their environment. While the United States has the highest rate of child poverty and one of the lowest rates of social mobility, it also spends the least on early childhood education, public health, and social services to support families. The report calls for greater attention to the needs of children and families, but it notes that certain US cultural and political values have been influential in limiting family support programs and government interventions to reduce the production and consumption of unhealthy foods, tobacco products, and guns. These values include "individual freedom," "free enterprise," "self-reliance," "federalism," and the "role of religion."

These are precisely the contested values that underlie the current ideological and partisan conflict over the role of the state in social policy, including the provision of health insurance to children. Thus, specific US social and political values and political structures contribute to policies that create the economic, social, and environmental risks to which children are exposed. These are the same values and structures that produced a children's health insurance program that is limited to certain categories of children, as well as a long, drawn-out political conflict over its reauthorization.

In the short term, the future of publicly funded children's coverage is related to a variety of implementation issues at the state level, including the commitment and capacity of states to enroll children and to insure the adequacy of health-care delivery within an environment of economic and fiscal uncertainty. One of the issues specific to the two different ways that children can be covered under the ACA is whether children will have to move back and forth between Medicaid or CHIP coverage and the health-insurance exchanges as family incomes change slightly (Thompson 2012: ch. 6). Within the child health policy community there continues to be concern about inequity in access and the quality of care that children receive. There are proposals for restructuring both funding and delivery systems in innovative ways (see Halfon, DuPlessis, and Inkelas 2007; Rosenbaum 2008) as well as proposals to reduce child poverty (for example, Bell, Bernstein, and Greenberg 2008; Mason and Kashen 2008).

But the longer-term future of children's access to care, the quality of that care, and whether the economic, social, and environmental causes of death and disease are reduced are intertwined with the future of both political and policy streams. The first question for predicting the future is whether Republicans or Democrats control Congress and the presidency; that outcome will dictate the extent to which federal monies are invested in programs that support families and children. Historically, Democrats have been far more willing to do that than have Republicans. Interviews conducted in 2010 by William Gormley Jr. with Democratic and Republican congressional committee staffers who worked on children's issues suggest that this will continue to be true. In their responses to a series of policy arguments about supporting children's programs, there is a very clear partisan divide (Gormley 2012: 127–130). One aspect of the politics of the Medicaid eligibility expansions in the late 1980s that is most striking from today's perspective is the bipartisan, trans-ideological support that developed through the efforts of the entrepreneurs of social learning (along with an agreement to separate the issues of children's health and abortion). Such a bipartisan policy consensus does not seem possible in the current extremely polarized world of US domestic policy.

The second question is whether the social medicine/public health paradigm reflected in *U.S. Health in International Perspective*, the 2013 report of the National Research Council and Institute of Medicine, moves from professional and academic policy networks to the political agenda—whether the kind of social learning around health services access that I describe here will be expanded to an integrated, interdisciplinary delivery system that attempts to improve the economic, social, and physical environments to which children are exposed. Serious action on this front will confront the ideological and structural barriers that to date have resulted in policies that separate people (and their children) into categories based on income. It is the historical maintenance of these walls against universalism in health and social policy that result in the comparative disadvantage suffered by US children.

Notes

1. William T. Gormley Jr. notes that other groups, such as the disabled and low-income elderly, are also viewed by the public as deserving of government and social resources (Gormley 2012: 5–6).

2. Beginning in the third quarter of 2004, two additional questions were added to the National Health Interview Survey (NHIS) insurance section to reduce potential errors in reporting Medicare and Medicaid status. Persons under age sixty-five with no reported coverage were asked explicitly about Medicaid coverage. Estimates of uninsurance for 2004 were calculated with the responses to these questions. Respondents who were reclassified as "covered" by the additional questions received the appropriate follow-up questions concerning periods of noncoverage for insured respondents. The two additional questions added beginning in the third quarter of 2004 did not affect the estimates of private coverage. Beginning in 2005, all estimates were calculated using this method. In 2006, NHIS underwent a sample redesign. The impact of the new sample design on estimates presented in this table is minimal.

3. This review and synthesis of existing research are major contributions to the policy literature on children's health insurance. Embry Howell and Genevieve Kenney note that "the research community has not yet come to agreement on the most appropriate methods for studying enrollment, access, use, and health status and experimentation continues on how best to conduct such studies. This is perhaps the greatest factor in the range of conclusions drawn from this comprehensive review of a diverse group of studies" (Howell and Kenney 2012: 390).

4. For discussions of the policy processes that resulted in the enactment of the ACA, see Starr (2011), McDonough (2011), Altman and Shactman (2011).

5. For some of the methodological limitations of the simulation, see Kenney et al. (2011).

6. HR 5652, The Sequester Replacement Reconciliation Act of 2012, introduced by Congressman Paul Ryan and HR 6684, The Spending Reduction Act of 2012, introduced by Congressman Eric Cantor. They also repealed other provisions of the ACA, including the establishment of health-insurance exchanges (Thomas.gov).

7. The House Select Committee on Children, Youth, and Families (1983–1993) held hearings and issued reports on health services for pregnant women and children in other nations; the National Commission to Prevent Infant Mortality published a booklet on "home visiting" in 1989 that described home visiting programs in other countries (National Commission to Prevent Infant Mortality 1989).

8. While infant mortality rates are clearly not a measure of the quality of children's health, these are a commonly used comparative measure because this information is collected in a more uniform way than are other measures.

9. Discussion of the comparative US infant mortality rate was analyzed in Chapter 2 as one aspect of the framing of the arguments for Medicaid eligibility expansions in the 1980s. The US infant mortality rate has continued to compare unfavorably with most other wealthy nations, and even with poorer nations (see MacDorman and Mathews 2010).

Acronyms

AAP	American Academy of Pediatrics
AARP	American Association of Retired Persons
ACA	Affordable Care Act
AFDC	Aid to Families with Dependent Children
AFL-CIO	American Federation of Labor and Congress of Industrial Organizations
AFSCME	American Federation of State, County, and Municipal Employees
AMA	American Medical Association
BBA	Balanced Budget Act
CCF	Center for Children and Families
CDF	Children's Defense Fund
CDHP	Children's Dental Health Project
CHAP	Child Health Assessment Program
CHC	community health center
CHILD	Child Health Insurance and Lower Deficit Act
CHIP	Children's Health Insurance Program
CHAMP	Children's Health and Medicare Protection Act
CHIPRA	Children's Health Insurance Program Reauthorization Act
CMS	Centers for Medicare and Medicaid Services
DHEW	Department of Health, Education, and Welfare
DHHS	Department of Health and Human Services
DPT	diphtheria-pertussis-tetanus
EPSDT	Early Periodic Screening, Diagnosis, and Treatment

FPL	federal poverty level
HMO	health maintenance organization
MACPAC	Medicaid and CHIP Payment and Access Commission
MCH	Maternal and Child Health
NACHRI	National Association of Children's Hospitals and Related Institutions
NCLR	National Council of La Raza
NGA	National Governors Association
NILC	National Immigration Law Center
OTA	Congressional Office of Technology Assessment
PhRMA	Pharmaceutical Research and Manufacturers of America
PPO	preferred provider organization
SCHIP	State Children's Health Insurance Program
SEIU	Service Employees International Union
UNICEF	United Nations Children's Fund
WIC	Women, Infants, and Children program

References

Abramowitz, Alan I. 2010. *The Disappearing Center.* New Haven, CT: Yale University Press.
Altenstetter, Christa, and James Warner Bjorkman. 1978. *Federal-State Health Policies and Impacts: The Politics of Implementation.* Washington, DC: University Press of America.
Altman, Stuart, and David Shactman. 2011. *Power, Politics, and Universal Health Care.* Amherst, NY: Prometheus Books.
American Academy of Pediatrics. 1993. "Child Health Financing Report." Washington, DC.
Bachrach, Peter, and Morton S. Baratz. 1970. *Power and Poverty, Theory and Practice.* New York: Oxford University Press.
Barone, Michael, and Grant Ujifusa. 1986. *The Almanac of American Politics.* Washington, DC: National Journal.
Barr, Sarah. 2008a. "SCHIP: House Democrats Criticize SCHIP Directive, Citing Negative Effects, Improper Procedures." *BNA Health Care Policy Report* (May 19).
———. 2008b. "Medicaid/SCHIP: Medicaid Funding, SCHIP Reauthorization Top Agenda for States, Safety-Net Providers." *BNA Health Care Policy Report* (November 17).
———. 2009a. "SCHIP: House Passes Reauthorization Funding to Expand Coverage to 4.1 Million Children." *BNA Health Care Policy Report* (January 19).
———. 2009b. "SCHIP: Senate Passes Reauthorization Bill After Rejecting GOP Efforts to Narrow Scope." *BNA Health Care Policy Report* (February 2).
Baumgartner, Frank R., and Bryan D. Jones. 1993. *Agendas and Instability in American Politics.* Chicago: University of Chicago Press.
Bell, Kate, Jared Bernstein, and Mark Greenberg. 2008. "Lessons for the United States from Other Advanced Economies in Tackling Child Poverty." In *Big Ideas for Children: Investing in Our Nation's Future,* 81–92. Washington, DC: First Focus.

Binder, Sarah A. 2001. "Congress, the Executive, and the Production of Public Policy: United We Govern?" In *Congress Reconsidered*, edited by Lawrence C. Dodd and Bruce I. Oppenheimer. Washington, DC: QC Press.

Birkland, Thomas A. 2010. *An Introduction to the Policy Process*. 3rd ed. New York: M. E. Sharpe.

Black, J. E. 1988. "The Sentimental Marketplace: Who Controls Child Health Care?" In *Money, Power and Health Care*, edited by Evan M. Melhado, Walter Feinberg, and Harold M. Swartz. Ann Arbor, MI: Health Administration Press.

BNA. 1996. "Massachusetts: Lawmakers Override Veto to Enact Plan to Expand Coverage to 170,000." *BNA Health Care Policy Report* (July 29).

———. 1997a. "Reform Proposals: Voters Divided on Health Care Issues, Children's Coverage Is Only Consensus." *BNA Health Care Policy Report* (January 27).

———. 1997b. "Children's Health: Lack of Consensus on Best Approach Blocks Kid Care from 'Common Agenda.'" *BNA Health Care Policy Report* (February 17).

———. 1997c. "Children's Health: Lott Suggests Unlimited MSA Program as One Way to Cover Uninsured Children." *BNA Health Care Policy Report* (April 14).

———. 1997d. "Children's Health: Senate Approach to Kid Care Favored by Hospital Officials, Advocacy Groups." *BNA Health Care Policy Report* (July 7).

———. 2006a. "SCHIP: States Face Shortfalls in FY2007, Looking Toward Congress for Solution." *BNA Health Care Policy Report* (February 27).

———. 2006b. "Health Savings Accounts/Waxman Challenges Insurance Industry to Stay Off White House 'HSA Bandwagon.'" *BNA Health Care Policy Report* (March 13).

———. 2006c. "SCHIP: As States Face Allotment Shortfalls, CRS Proposes Options for Fixing Imbalance." *BNA Health Care Policy Report* (April 24).

———. 2006d. "SCHIP: Stakeholders Propose Improvements as Congressional Reauthorization Nears." *BNA Health Care Policy Report* (June 26).

———. 2006e. "SCHIP: Children's Coverage at Risk If Program Not Funded Adequately, States Tell Congress." *BNA Health Care Policy Report* (December 4).

———. 2006f. "SCHIP: Health Groups Urge Quick Reauthorization, Additional Funds for Child Health Program." *BNA Health Care Policy Report* (December 18).

———. 2007a. "SCHIP: Senators to Move Quickly on Reauthorization; Rockefeller Predicts Enactment of SCHIP Bill." *BNA Health Care Policy Report* (January 22).

———. 2007b. "SCHIP: House, Senate Pass Budget Resolution; Tobacco Tax Increase for SCHIP Left Out." *BNA Health Care Policy Report* (May 21).

———. 2007c. "SCHIP: NGA Urges Congress to Maintain State Flexibility on SCHIP Coverage Options." *BNA Health Care Policy Report* (June 18).

———. 2007d. "SCHIP: Most Americans Support Tobacco Tax Hike to Help Finance SCHIP, Opinion Poll Shows." *BNA Health Care Policy Report* (June 25).

———. 2007e. "SCHIP: Democrats Take Aim at Study Estimating That Only 700,000 Eligible Kids Not Enrolled." *BNA Health Care Policy Report* (June 25).

———. 2007f. "SCHIP: Senate Finance Republicans Ask Bush to Stop Approving Waivers to Cover Adults." *BNA Health Care Policy Report* (July 16).

———. 2007g. "Reform Proposals: Health Care Coalition Releases Agenda Calling for Less Government Involvement." *BNA Health Care Policy Report* (July 23).

———. 2007h. "Governors, Health Officials Seek Withdrawal of CMS Rules Targeting 'Crowd-Out' by SCHIP." *BNA Health Care Policy Report* (September 10).

———. 2007i. "Senators Ask Bush to Rescind Controversial 'Crowd-Out' Policy." *BNA Health Care Policy Report* (September 17).

———. 2007j. "Senators Introduce Bill to Block CMS from Implementing Enrollment Restrictions." *BNA Health Care Policy Report* (September 17).

———. 2008a. "Congress: House Speaker Touts Biomedical Research, Mental Health Parity, Children's Health Bills." *BNA Health Care Policy Report* (January 28).

———. 2008b. "Connecticut, Massachusetts AGs Support Lawsuit Seeking to Block SCHIP Restrictions." *BNA Health Care Policy Report* (April 14).

———. 2008c. "SCHIP: Authority for CMS to Issue Directive Limiting Enrollment Debated at Hearing." *BNA Health Care Policy Report* (April 14).

———. 2008d. "With Resolution Markup Stymied, Democrats Vow to Continue Fight Against Bush Policy." *BNA Health Care Policy Report* (July 28).

———. 2008e. "Senator Baucus Welcomes CMS Decision Not to Enforce Controversial SCHIP Directive." *BNA Health Care Policy Report* (August 25).

———. 2009. "Medicaid/SCHIP: Future of Safety-Net Programs Depends on Congressional Efforts to Shore Up Funding." *BNA Health Care Policy Report* (January 19).

Brandon, William P., Rosemary V. Chaudry, and Alice Sardell. 2001. "Launching SCHIP: The States and Children's Health Insurance." In *The New Politics of State Health Policy,* edited by Robert Hackey and David Rochefort. Lawrence: University Press of Kansas.

Brooks, Tricia. 2009. "New CHIPRA Dental Standards: A Victory for Kids!" Georgetown University Center for Children and Families, A Children's Health Blog. http://ccf.georgetown.edu/ccf-resources/new_chipra_dental_standards_a_victory_for_kids.

Burns, Carole. 1997. "States Acting on Child Health Care." *New York Times*, May 26.

CCF. 2007a. "Summary of the House SCHIP Bill: Children's Health and Medicare Protection Act of 2007 (CHAMP Act)." Center for Children and Families, Georgetown University Health Policy Institute. http/www.ccf.georgetown.edu/index/cms-filesystem-action?file=ccf&20publication/federal.

———. 2007b. "Summary of the Senate SCHIP Bill: The Children's Health Insurance Program Reauthorization Act of 2007." Center for Children and Families, Georgetown University Health Policy Institute. http/www.ccf.georgetown.edu/index/cms-filesystem-action?file=ccf&20publication/federal.

———. 2009. "The Children's Health Insurance Program Reauthorization Act of 2009, Overview and Summary." March. http://ccf.georgetown.edu/wp-content/uploads/2012/03/chip-summary-03-09.pdf.

———. 2012. "CHIPRA at Work Three Years Later: Shaping State Actions and Connecting Children to Coverage." February. http://ccf.georgetown.edu/ccf-resources/chipra-at-work-three-years-later-shaping-state-actions-and-connecting-children-to-coverage-2/.

Children's Access to Health Coverage: Hearing Before the Subcomm. on Health of the H. Comm. on Ways and Means, 105th Cong. (April 8, 1997).

Children's Dental Health Project. 2010. "Oral Health Provisions Included in the Children's Health Insurance Program Reauthorization Act of 2009 (CHIPRA)." February. http://www.cdhp.org/resource_types/presentations.
Children's Health Insurance Program in Action: A State's Perspective on CHIP: Hearing Before the S. Comm. on Fin., 110th Cong. (April 4, 2007).
CHIP at 10: A Decade of Covering Children: Hearing Before the Subcomm. on Health Care of the S. Comm. on Finance, 109th Cong. (July 25, 2006).
CHIP Program from the States' Perspective: Hearing Before the Subcomm. on Health Care of the S. Comm. on Fin., 109th Cong. (November 16, 2006).
Chong, Dennis, and James Druckman. 2007. "Framing Theory." *Annual Review of Political Science* 10: 103–126.
Cigler, Beverly A. 2011. "Not Just Another Special Interest: The Intergovernmental Lobby Revisited." In *Interest Group Politics*, edited by Allan J. Cigler and Burdett A. Loomis. Washington, DC: CQ Press.
Cloud, David S. 1994. "Support Erodes as Key Backers Voice Little Hope for Passage." *Congressional Quarterly* (September 17): 2571–2572.
Clymer, Adam. 1999. *Edward M. Kennedy: A Biography.* New York: William Morrow.
Cobb, Roger W., and Charles Elder. 1983. *Participation in American Politics: The Dynamics of Agenda-Building.* Baltimore, MD: Johns Hopkins University Press.
Cobb, Roger W., and Marc Howard Ross, eds. 1997. *Cultural Strategies of Agenda Denial.* Lawrence: University Press of Kansas.
Cohen, Richard E. 1998. "Congress: Business as Usual." *National Journal* (March 7). http://assets.nationaljournal.com//voteratings/historical/1997_VoteRatings _Cover_Story.pdf.
Cohen, Sally S. 2001. *Championing Child Care.* New York: Columbia University Press.
Committee for Economic Development. 1987. *Children in Need: Investment Strategies for the Educationally Disadvantaged.* New York: Committee for Economic Development.
Committee on Energy and Commerce. 2007. "Dingell, Clinton Announce Initiative to Expand Access to Healthcare Coverage to All Children." News Release. March 14.
Coughlin, Teresa A., Leighton Ku, and John Holahan. 1994. *Medicaid Since 1980: Costs, Coverage and the Shifting Alliances Between the Federal Government and the States.* Washington, DC: The Urban Institute Press.
Covering the Uninsured Through the Eyes of a Child: Hearing Before the Subcomm. on Health of the H. Comm. on Energy and Commerce, 110th Cong. (February 14 and March 1, 2007).
Covering Uninsured Children: The Impact of the August 17 CHIP Directive: Hearing Before the Subcomm. on Health of the S. Comm. on Fin., 110th Cong. (April 9, 2008).
Covering Uninsured Kids: Missed Opportunities for Moving Forward: Hearing Before the Subcomm. on Health of the H. Comm. on Energy and Commerce, 110th Cong. (January 29, 2008).
Covering Uninsured Kids: Reversing Progress Already Made: Hearing Before the H. Comm. on Energy and Commerce, 110th Cong. (February 26 and 28, 2008).
Crowley, Jocelyn Elise. 2003. *The Politics of Child Support in America.* Cambridge, UK: Cambridge University Press.

Davidson, Roger H., and Walter J. Oleszek. 2002. *Congress and Its Members*. 8th ed. Washington, DC: CQ Press.

Davis, Karen, and Cathy Schoen. 1978. *Health and the War on Poverty*. Washington, DC: The Brookings Institution.

DeParle, Jason. 1993. "Advocates Sell Antipoverty Policies Beneath Faces of America's Children." *New York Times*, March 29.

DHHS. 2012. "Child Health USA 2012." Health Resources and Services Administration, Maternal and Child Health Bureau, Rockville, MD.

Dionne, E. J., Jr. 1987. "Children Emerge as an Issue for Democrats." *New York Times*, September 27.

Edelstein, Burton L. 2009. "Putting Teeth in CHIP: 1997–2009 Retrospective of Congressional Action on Children's Oral Health." *Academic Pediatrics* 9 (6): 467–475.

Executive Business Meeting to Consider Adoption of the Committee's Rules for the 111th Congress and an Original Bill Reauthorizing the Children's Health Insurance Program: Hearing Before the S. Comm. on Fin., 111th Cong. (January 15, 2009).

Families USA. 2003a. "Covering Pregnant Women: CHIPRA Offers a New Option." Washington, DC. http://www.familiesusa.org/assets/pdfs/chipra/Covering-Pregnant-Women.pdf.

———. 2003b. "The Immigrant Children's Health Improvement Act (ICHIA): A Good Investment in America's Future." Fact Sheet. Washington, DC. http://www.familiesusa.org/assets/pdfs/ICHIA_Good_Investment_Dec_11_200 37965.pdf.

Federal Interagency Forum on Child and Family Health. 2012. "America's Children in Brief 2012: Key National Indicators of Well-Being." http://childstats.gov/pdf/ac2101/ac_12.pdf.

Federal Register. 1997. "Annual Update of the HHS Poverty Guidelines." 62 (46): 10856–10859. March 10. http://aspe.hhs.gov/poverty/97fedreg.htm.

First Focus. 2008. *Big Ideas for Children*. Washington, DC: First Focus.

———. 2013. "Child Health: What the Passage of Health Reform Means for Children." http://firstfocus.net/sites/default/files/HealthReformPassage.pdf.

Foltz, Anne-Marie. 1982. *An Ounce of Prevention: Child Health Policy Under Medicaid*. Cambridge, MA: MIT Press.

Ford Foundation. 1989. *The Common Good, Social Welfare and the American Future*. New York: Ford Foundation Project on Social Welfare and the American Future.

The Future of CHIP: Improving the Health of America's Children: Hearing Before the S. Comm. on Fin., 110th Cong. (February 1, 2007).

Galvin, Robert. 2007. "Consumerism and Controversy: A Conversation with Regina Hertzlinger." *Health Affairs* 26: 552–559.

Glasow, Richard D. 1986. *School-Based Clinics, the Abortion Connection*. Washington, DC: National Right to Life Educational Trust Fund.

Goggin, Malcolm L. 1987. *Policy Design and the Politics of Implementation: The Case of Child Health Care in the American States*. Knoxville: University of Tennessee Press.

Gormley, William T., Jr. 1995. *Everybody's Children: Child Care as a Public Problem*. Washington, DC: The Brookings Institution.

———. 2010. "Arguing for Kids: Issue Framing Effects." Paper presented at the Annual Meeting of the American Political Science Association, Washington, DC, September 3.

———. 2012. *Voices for Children: Rhetoric and Public Policy*. Washington, DC: Brookings Institution Press.

Government Accounting Office (GAO). 1996. *Health Insurance for Children: Private Insurance Continues to Deteriorate*. GAO/HEHS-96-129.

Governors' Perspective on Medicaid: Hearing Before the S. Comm. on Fin., 105th Cong. (March 11, 1997).

Grason, Holly, and Bernard Guyer. 1995. "Rethinking the Organization of Children's Programs: Lessons from the Elderly." *Milbank Quarterly* 73 (4): 565–597.

Grogan, Colleen, and Eric Patashnik. 2003. "Between Welfare Medicine and Mainstream Entitlement: Medicaid at the Political Crossroads." *Journal of Health Politics, Policy and Law* 28 (5): 821–858.

Gutterman, David S. 2002. "Innocence, or, To God and Country, Home and Mall and Most of All—for the Children." Paper prepared for the Meeting of the American Political Science Association, Boston, MA, August 29–September 1.

Hacker, Jacob S. 2002. *The Divided Welfare State: The Battle over Public and Private Benefits in the U.S.* New York: Cambridge University Press.

Halfon, Neal, Helen DuPlessis, and Moira Inkelas. 2007. "Transforming the U.S. Child Health System." *Health Affairs* 26 (2): 315–330.

Halpern, Sydney A. 1988. *American Pediatrics: The Social Dynamics of Professionalism, 1880–1980*. Berkeley: University of California Press.

Harkin, Tom. 1994. "News Release from the Office of Senator Tom Harkin." September 14.

Health Insurance for Pregnant Women and Children: Hearing Before the Subcomm. on Health of the H. Comm. on Ways and Means, 101st Cong. (March 20, 1990).

Heritage Foundation. 2007a. "SCHIP and 'Crowd-Out': The High Cost of Expanding Eligibility," WebMemo no. 1518, June 21.

———. 2007b. "SCHIP and 'Crowd-Out': How Public Program Expansion Reduces Coverage," WebMemo no. 31627, September 19.

Himelfarb, Richard. 1995. *Catastrophic Politics: The Rise and Fall of the Medicare Catastrophic Coverage Act of 1988*. University Park: Pennsylvania State University Press.

Holahan, John. 1997. *Expanding Insurance Coverage for Children*. Washington, DC: The Urban Institute.

Hosansky, David. 1997. "Health: Concern for Uninsured Children Has Not Led to Agreement." *CQ Weekly* (April): 850.

Howell, Embry M., and Genevieve M. Kenney. 2012. "The Impact of the Medicaid/CHIP Expansions on Children: A Synthesis of the Evidence." *Medical Care Research and Review* 69 (4): 372–396.

HR 5998 Protecting Children's Health Coverage of 2008: Hearing Before the Subcomm. on Health of the H. Comm. on Energy and Commerce, 110th Cong. (May 15, 2008).

Hutchins, Vince L. 1997. "A History of Child Health and Pediatrics in the United States." In *Health Care for Children*, edited by Ruth E. K. Stein, 79–196. New York: United Hospital Fund of New York.

Iglehart, John K. 2007a. "Insuring All Children—the New Political Imperative." *New England Journal of Medicine* 357 (1) (July 5): 70–76.

———. 2007b. "The Fate of SCHIP—Surrogate Marker for Health Care Ideology?" *New England Journal of Medicine* 357 (21) (November 22): 2104–2107.

———. 2009a. "Dental Coverage in SCHIP: The Legacy of Deamonte Driver." Health Affairs Blog. January 30. http://healthaffairs.org/blog/2009/01/30/dental-coverage-in-schip-the-legacy-of-deamonte-driver/.

———. 2009b. "Expanding Coverage for Children—the Democrats' Power and SCHIP Reauthorization." *New England Journal of Medicine* 360 (9) (February 26): 855–857.

Imig, Doug. 1996. "Advocacy by Proxy: The Children's Lobby in American Politics." *Journal of Children and Poverty* 2: 31–53.

———. 2001. "Mobilizing Parents and Communities for Children." In *Who Speaks for America's Children? The Role of Child Advocates in Public Policy,* edited by Carol J. DeVita and Rachel Mosher-Williams, 191–207. Washington, DC: The Urban Institute Press.

———. 2006. "Building a Social Movement for America's Children." *Journal of Children and Poverty* 12 (1): 21–37.

Improving the Health Status of Children: Hearing Before S. Comm. on Labor and Human Resources, 105th Cong. (April 18, 1997).

Inside Dentistry. 2011. "The Einstein Series: A Conversation with Burton L. Edelstein." *Inside Dentistry* 7 (April).

Institute of Medicine and National Research Council. 2011. "Child and Adolescent Health and Health Care Quality: Measuring What Matters." Washington, DC. http://www.nap.edu/catalog.php?record_id=13084.

Insuring Bright Futures: Improving Access to Dental Care and Providing a Healthy Start for Children: Hearing Before the Subcomm. on Health of the H. Comm. on Energy and Commerce, 110th Cong. (March 27, 2007).

Jacobs, Lawrence R. 1993. *The Health of Nations: Public Opinion and the Making of American and British Health Policy.* Ithaca, NY: Cornell University Press.

Johnson, Kay A. 1999. "Breaking Away: Advocacy, Education, and the Relationship Between Maternal and Child Health Professionals and the American Public Health Association." *Maternal and Child Health Journal* 3 (1): 53–60.

Johnson, Kay A., Chris DeGraw, Colleen Sonosky, Anne Markus, and Sara Rosenbaum. 1997. "Children's Health Insurance: A Comparison of Major Federal Legislation." Report from the Center for Health Policy Research. Washington, DC: The George Washington University Medical Center.

Johnson, Kay, Dana Hughes, and Sara Rosenbaum. 1988. "Advocacy for Women and Children." In *Maternal and Child Health Practices,* edited by Helen M. Wallace, George M. Ryan, and Allan C. Olgelsby, 203–213. Oakland, CA: Third Party Publishers.

Johnson, Kay A., and John E. McDonough. 1998. *Expanding Health Coverage for Children: Matching Federal Policies and State Strategies.* New York: Milbank Memorial Fund.

Kaiser Family Foundation. 2012a. "Children and Oral Health: Assessing Needs, Coverage and Access." Kaiser Commission on Medicaid and the Uninsured Issue Brief, June 12. http://kaiserfamilyfoundation.files.wordpress.com/2013/01/7681-04.pdf.

———. 2012b. "Health Coverage of Children: The Role of Medicaid and CHIP." Kaiser Commission on Medicaid and the Uninsured Fact Sheet. July. www.kff.org/uninsured/upload/7698-06.pdf.

———. 2013. "Status of State Action on the Medicaid Expansion Decision, as of October 22, 2013." Chart. http://kff.org/health-reform/state-indicator/state-activity-around-expanding-medicaid-under-the-affordable-care-act/.

Katz, Michael B. 1983. *Poverty and Policy in American History*. New York: Academic Press.
Kenney, Genevieve M., Matthew Buettgens, Jocelyn Guyer, and Martha Heberlein. 2011. "Improving Coverage for Children Under Health Reform Will Require Maintaining Current Eligibility Standards." *Health Affairs* 30 (12): 2371–2381.
Kingdon, John W. 1995. *Agendas, Alternatives, and Public Policies*. 2nd ed. New York: HarperCollins.
Knox, Richard A. 1994. "U.S. Children Focus of New Health Bid." *Boston Globe*, September 12.
Kosterlitz, Julie. 1986a. "Split over Pregnancy." *National Journal* (June 21): 1538–1541.
———. 1986b. "Concern About Children." *National Journal* (September 20): 2255–2258.
———. 1986c. "Children's Agenda Making Headway in States." *National Journal* (November 22): 2849.
———. 1989. "Watch Out for Waxman." *National Journal* (March 11): 577–581.
Lesley, Bruce. 2008. Testimony before the Subcommittee on Health, House Committee on Energy and Commerce, "Covering Uninsured Kids: Missed Opportunities for Moving Forward." January 29.
MacDorman, Marian F., and T. J. Mathews. 2010. "Behind International Rankings of Infant Mortality: How the U.S. Compares with Europe." *International Journal of Health Services* 40 (4): 577–588.
Mann, Cindy. 2007. Testimony Submitted to the Senate Committee on Finance Hearing, "The Future of CHIP: Improving the Health of America's Children." February 1.
Mann, Thomas E., and Norman J. Orenstein. 2012. *It's Even Worse Than It Looks: How the American Constitutional System Collided with the New Politics of Extremism*. New York: Basic Books.
Marieskind, H. I. 1980. *Women in the Health System: Patients, Providers and Programs*. St. Louis, MO: C. V. Mosby.
Markus, Anne R. 1996. "Children's Continuity of Coverage Under the Kassebaum-Kennedy Bill." In *Health Policy and Child Health*. Washington, DC: Center for Health Policy Research, George Washington University Medical Center.
Marlow, G. R. 1995. "A Voice for the Voteless: Moral Themes and the 'Language of Good' in the Rhetoric of Marian Wright Edelman." PhD diss., University of Kansas, Lawrence.
Marmor, Theodore R. 1983. "Rethinking National Health Insurance." In *Political Analysis and American Medical Care, Essays*. Cambridge, UK: Cambridge University Press.
———. 2000. *The Politics of Medicare*. New York: Aldine De Gruyter.
Marshner, Connie, and Nina Owcharenko. 2007. "The State Children's Health Insurance Program: High Stakes for American Families." *The Heritage Foundation*, WebMemo no. 1528, June 27. www.heritage.org/research/reports/2007/06/the-state-childrens-health-insurance-pro.
Mason, Elisabeth, and Julie Kashen. 2008. "Out of the Desert: An Integrated Approach to Ending Child Poverty." In *Big Ideas for Children: Investing in Our Nation's Future*, 25–29. Washington, DC: First Focus.
Mayall, Berry. 1998. "Towards a Sociology of Child Health." *Sociology of Health and Illness* 20 (3): 269–288.
McDonough, John E. 2000. *Experiencing Politics*. Berkeley: University of California Press.

———. 2011. *Inside National Health Reform*. Berkeley: University of California Press and Milbank Memorial Fund.

Meckler, Laura. 2009. "Children's Health Bill Aids Legal Immigrants." *Wall Street Journal*, January 13.

Morone, James A. 2003. *Hellfire Nation: The Politics of Sin in American History*. New Haven, CT: Yale University Press.

Morone, James A., E. H. Kilbreth, and K. M. Langwell. 2001. "Back to School: A Health Care Strategy for Youth." *Health Affairs* 20 (1): 122–136.

NACHRI. 1992. *About NACHRI*. October. Obtained by the author from Professor Craig Ramsay, Ohio Wesleyan University.

Nather, David. 1996. "Reform Proposals: Few Easy Issues Remain After Passage of Incremental Health Reform Package." *BNA Health Care Policy Report* (August 12).

———. 1997a. "U.S. Budget: Clinton Budget Revives Medicaid Caps, Proposes Limited Health Plan for Kids." *BNA Health Care Policy Report* (February 10).

———. 1997b. "Medicaid: Clinton Proposal Draws Mixed Reviews; Caps Worry Providers, Some Republicans." *BNA Health Care Policy Report* (February 17).

———. 1997c. "U.S. Budget: Congress Approves Budget Resolution as Work Begins on Health Legislation." *BNA Health Care Policy Report* (June 9).

———. 1997d. "Children's Health: Thomas Plans to Include Tax Incentives for Kid Care in Ways and Means Package." *BNA Health Care Policy Report* (June 9).

———. 1997e. "U.S. Budget: Commerce Approves Medicaid, Kid Care After Restoring Repeal of the Boren Law." *BNA Health Care Policy Report* (June 16).

———. 1997f. "Medicaid: Finance Clears Medicaid Kid Care, Expands Funding for Children's Coverage." *BNA Health Care Policy Report* (June 23).

———. 1997g. "Children's Health: Kennedy Effort to Boost Tobacco Tax for Kid Coverage Defeated by Senate." *BNA Health Care Policy Report* (July 7).

———. 1997h. "U.S. Budget: NGA Endorses House Kid Care Plan as Groups Push Senate Version." *BNA Health Care Policy Report* (July 14).

———. 1997i. "U.S. Budget: GOP Divided over Kid Benefits: Choice of Seven Plans Under Discussion." *BNA Health Care Policy Report* (July 21).

———. 1997j. "Children's Health: Health Care Becomes Reality in Compromise Plan." *BNA Health Care Policy Report* (August 4).

———. 1997k. "Medicaid: Agreement Clears Way for Flexibility, Walks Fine Line on DSH Funding." *BNA Health Care Policy Report* (August 4).

Nather, David, and Alexis Simendinger. 1997. "Children's Health: Daschle to Introduce Tax Subsidy Plan, Will Follow Debate on Other Approaches." *BNA Health Care Policy Report* (January 13).

Nather, David, and Steve Teske. 1997a. "U.S. Budget: Senate Averts Kids' Health Trouble, While House Approves Budget Resolution." *BNA Health Care Policy Report* (May 26).

———. 1997b. "U.S. Budget: Finance Committee Draft Hints at Plans for Health Savings, Children's Coverage." *BNA Health Care Policy* Report (June 16).

———. 1997c. "U.S. Budget: Senate, House Clear Budget Packages After Changing Kid's Care, Medicaid Plans." *BNA Health Care Policy* Report (June 30).

National Commission on Children. 1991. *Beyond Rhetoric: A New American Agenda for Children and Families*. Washington, DC: US Government Printing Office.

National Commission to Prevent Infant Mortality. 1988. *Death Before Life: The Tragedy of Infant Mortality*. Washington, DC.

———. 1989. *Home Visiting: Opening Doors for America's Pregnant Women and Children.* Washington, DC.
National Immigration Law Center. 2007. "NILC Urges Congress to Honor Its Commitment to Immigrant Children." September 28. www.nilc.org/immspbs/cdev/ICHIA/ichia002.htm.
Nelson, Thomas E., Dana E. Wittmer, and Allyson F. Shortle. 2010. "Framing and Value Recruitment in the Debate over Teaching Evolution." In *Winning with Words: The Origins and Impact of Political Framing,* edited by Brian F. Schaffner and Patrick J. Sellers, 11–40. New York: Routledge.
New York Times. 1997. "Insuring Children, Sensibly." April 8.
Noah, Timothy. 1991. "Governors, Harried by Medicaid Costs, Point Their Fingers at Rep. Waxman." *Wall Street Journal,* February 4.
Oberg, C. N., and C. L. Polich. 1988. "Medicaid: Entering the Third Decade." *Health Affairs* 7 (4): 83–96.
Oberlander, Jonathan. 1995. "Families USA (United for Senior Action) Foundation." In *U.S. Health Policy Groups: Institutional Profiles,* edited by Craig Ramsay, 209–212. Westport, CT: Greenwood Press.
———. 2003. *The Political Life of Medicare.* Chicago: University of Chicago Press.
Oberlander, Jonathan B., and Barbara Lyons. 2009. "Beyond Incrementalism: SCHIP and the Politics of Health Reform." *Health Affairs* 28 (3): 399–410. doi: 10.1377/hlthaff.28.3.w399.
Oliver, Thomas, and Pamela Paul-Shaheen. 1997. "Translating Ideas into Action: Entrepreneurial Leadership in State Health Care Reform." *Journal of Health Politics, Policy and Law* 22 (3): 721–788.
Olson, Laura Katz. 2010. *The Politics of Medicaid.* New York: Columbia University Press.
Open Executive Session to Consider the CHIP Reauthorization Act of 2007: Hearing Before S. Comm. on Fin., 110th Cong. (July 19, 2007).
Oregonian. 1997. "Fouling the Air." May 15.
OTA (Office of Technology Assessment, US Congress). 1988. *Healthy Children: Investing in the Future.*
Otto, Mary. 2007. "Boy's Death Fuels Drives to Fund Dental Aid to Poor." *Washington Post,* March 7. http://www.washingtonpost.com/wp-dyn/content/article/2007/03/02/AR2007030200827.html.
Owcharenko, Nina. 2007. Testimony Submitted to the Health Subcommittee of the House Committee on Energy and Commerce Hearing, "Covering the Uninsured Through the Eyes of a Child." February 14.
Pear, Robert. 1990. "Deficit or No Deficit, Unlikely Allies Bring About Expansion in Medicaid." *New York Times,* November 4.
———. 1991. "Agreement on Health Care Eludes Panel." *New York Times,* December 3.
———. 1994. "Clintons Should Address Health Care One Issue at a Time, Experts Suggest." *New York Times,* October 10.
———. 1997a. "President Moves to Protect Half of Uninsured Children." *New York Times,* February 7.
———. 1997b. "Hatch Joins Kennedy to Back a Health Program." *New York Times,* March 14.
———. 1997c. "Closest to Their Hearts." *New York Times,* July 29.
———. 2007. "A Battle over Expansion of Children's Health Insurance." *New York Times,* July 9.

———. 2009. "Congress Set to Renew Health Care for Children." *New York Times*, January 13.
Pear, Robert, and Carl Hulse. 2007. "Immigrant Bill Dies in Senate; Defeat for Bush." *New York Times*, June 29.
Peterson, Mark A. 1993. "Political Influence in the 1990s: From Iron Triangles to Policy Networks." *Journal of Health Politics, Policy and Law* 18 (2): 395–438.
———. 1995. "How Health Policy Information Is Used in Congress." In *Intensive Care: How Congress Shapes Health Policy,* edited by Thomas E. Mann and Norman J. Ornstein. Washington, DC: American Enterprise Institute and Brookings Institution.
———. 1997. "The Limits of Social Learning: Translating Analysis into Action." *Journal of Health Politics, Policy and Law* 22 (4): 1077–1114.
Pierson, Paul. 1992. "'Policy Feedbacks' and Political Change: Contrasting Reagan and Thatcher's Pension-Reform Initiatives." *Studies in American Political Development* 6: 359–390.
———. 2000. "Increasing Returns, Path Dependence, and the Study of Politics." *American Political Science Review* 9 (2): 241–267.
Quadagno, Jill. 2005. *One Nation Uninsured: Why the U.S. Has No National Health Insurance.* New York: Oxford University Press.
Ramsay, Craig. 1995a. "American Academy of Pediatrics (AAP)." In *U.S. Health Policy Groups: Institutional Profiles,* edited by Craig Ramsay, 19–21. Westport, CT: Greenwood Press.
———. 1995b. "March of Dimes Birth Defects Foundation (MDBDF)." In *U.S. Health Policy Groups: Institutional Profiles,* edited by Craig Ramsay, 268–270. Westport, CT: Greenwood Press.
———. 1995c. "National Governors' Association (NGA)." In *U.S. Health Policy Groups: Institutional Profiles,* edited by Craig Ramsay, 336–341. Westport, CT: Greenwood Press.
Richmond, Linda Micco. 2006. "SCHIP: GOP Senator Urges Boost in SCHIP Funding, but States Question Federal Support Formula." *BNA Health Care Policy Report* (December 4).
———. 2007a. "SCHIP Reauthorization, Medicaid, Pharmaceuticals Viewed as Legislative Priorities." *BNA Health Care Policy Report* (January 15).
———. 2007b. "SCHIP: Senate Considers Funding, Flexibility in First SCHIP Reauthorization Hearing." *BNA Health Care Policy Report* (February 5).
———. 2007c. "Access: House Panel Debates Tax Credits, Income, Coverage of Adults Under Children's Program." *BNA Health Care Policy Report* (February 26).
Roberts, Steven V. 1983. "Now a Select Committee for Families." *New York Times*, February 23.
Rochefort, David A., and Roger W. Cobb, eds. 1994. *The Politics of Problem Definition: Shaping the Policy Agenda.* Lawrence: University Press of Kansas.
Rosenbaum, Sara. 1988. "Lives in the Balance." Unpublished manuscript.
———. 2008. "Cutting the Gordian Knot: National Reforms to Assure Coverage of Developmental Child Health Treatment." In *Big Ideas for Children: Investing in Our Nation's Future,* 129–136. Washington, DC: First Focus.
Rosenbaum, Sara, and Colleen A. Sonosky. 2001. "Medicaid Reforms and SCHIP: Health Care Coverage and the Changing Policy Environment." In *Who Speaks for America's Children? The Role of Child Advocates in Public Policy,* edited by Carol J. DeVita and Rachel Mosher-Williams. Washington, DC: The Urban Institute Press.

Rovner, Julie. 1989. "Health/Human Services: Impasse over Deficit Bill Snags Social Initiatives." *Congressional Quarterly Weekly Report* (October 31): 800–801.

Rowley, Diane L., Theresa Chapple-McGruder, Dara D. Mendez, and Dorothy Browne. 2013. "Disparities in Maternal and Child Health in the United States." In *Maternal and Child Health: Programs, Problems and Policy in Public Health*, 3rd ed., edited by Jonathan B. Kotch, 233–253. Burlington, MA: Jones and Bartlett Learning.

Rubin, Alissa J., and David S. Cloud. 1994. "Doubt Surfaces on Bill Passage as Senate Struggle Continues." *Congressional Quarterly* (August 20): 2458–2460.

Ryan, Jennifer M. 2003. "SCHIP Turns 5: Taking Stock, Moving Ahead." In *The Nation's Health*, 7th ed., edited by Philip R. Lee and Carroll L. Estes, 428–438. Sudbury, MA: Jones and Bartlett.

Sabatier, Paul A. 1988. "An Advocacy Coalition Framework of Policy Change and the Role of Policy-Oriented Learning Therein." *Policy Sciences* 2: 129–168.

Sabatier, Paul A., and Hank C. Jenkins-Smith. 1999. "The Advocacy Coalition Framework: An Assessment." In *Theories of the Policy Process*, edited by Paul A. Sabatier, 117–166. Boulder, CO: Westview Press.

Sabatier, Paul A., and Christopher M. Weible. 2007. "The Advocacy Coalition Framework, Innovations and Clarifications." In *Theories of the Policy Process*, 2nd ed., edited by Paul A. Sabatier, 189–220. Boulder, CO: Westview Press.

Sardell, Alice. 1988. *The U.S. Experiment in Social Medicine: The Community Health Center Program, 1965–1986*. Pittsburgh, PA: The University of Pittsburgh Press.

———. 1991. "Child Health Policy in the U.S.: The Paradox of Consensus." In *Health Policy and the Disadvantaged*, edited by Lawrence D. Brown. Durham, NC: Duke University Press.

———. 1995. "The Children's Defense Fund." In *U.S. Women's Interest Groups: Institutional Profiles*, edited by Sarah Slavin, 112–115. Westport, CT: Greenwood Press.

———. 2012. "Community Health Centers: Successful Advocacy for Expanding Health Care Access." In *Politics and Policy in Nursing and Health Care*, 6th ed., edited by Diana Mason, Judith Leavitt, and Mary Chaffee. St. Louis, MO: Elsevier Science.

Sardell, Alice, and Kay Johnson. 1998. "The Politics of EPSDT in the 1990s: Policy Entrepreneurs, Political Streams, and Children's Health Benefits." *Milbank Quarterly* 76 (2): 175–205.

Schaffner, Brian F., and Patrick J. Sellers, eds. 2010. *Winning with Words: The Origins and Impact of Political Framing*. New York: Routledge.

Schattschneider, E. E. (1960) 1975. *The Semisovereign People: A Realist's View of Democracy in America*. New York: Holt, Rhinehart and Winston. Reprint, Hindsdale, IL: Dryden Press.

Schneider, Anne, and Helen Ingram. 1993. "Social Construction of Target Populations: Implications for Politics and Policy." *American Political Science Review* 87 (2): 334–347.

Serafini, Marilyn Werber. 1997. "Kidnapped." *National Journal* (March 22).

Skocpol, Theda. 1992. *Protecting Soldiers and Mothers*. Cambridge, MA: Harvard University Press.

———. 1997. *Boomerang: Health Care Reform and the Turn Against Government*. New York: W. W. Norton.

Skocpol, Theda, and Jillian Dickert. 2001. "Speaking for Children and Families in a Changing Civic America." In *Who Speaks for America's Children? The Role of Child Advocates in Public Policy,* edited by Carol J. DeVita and Rachel Mosher-Williams, 137–164. Washington, DC: The Urban Institute Press.

Smith, David G. 2002. *Entitlement Politics: Medicare and Medicaid, 1995–2001.* New York: Aldine de Gruyter.

Sommers, Anna, Stephen Zuckerman, Lisa Dubay, and Genevieve Kenney. 2007. "Substitution of SCHIP for Private Coverage: Results from a 2002 Evaluation in Ten States." *Health Affairs* 26 (2): 529–537.

Southern Regional Task Force on Infant Mortality. 1985. *Final Report for the Children of Tomorrow.* Washington, DC: Southern Regional Project on Infant Mortality.

Staff of H. Select Comm. on Children, Youth, and Families, 100th Cong. 1988. *Children and Families: Key Trends in the 1980s.*

Starfield, Barbara. 1985. "Motherhood and Apple Pie: The Effectiveness of Medical Care for Children." *Milbank Memorial Fund Quarterly* 63 (3): 523–546.

Starr, Paul. 2011. *Remedy and Reaction: The Peculiar American Struggle over Health Care Reform.* New Haven, CT: Yale University Press.

Stein, Ruth E. K., ed. 1997. *Health Care for Children.* New York: United Hospital Fund of New York.

Steiner, Gilbert Y. 1976. *The Children's Cause.* Washington, DC: The Brookings Institution.

Stevens, Robert, and Rosemary Stevens. 1974. *Welfare Medicine in America: A Case Study of Medicaid.* New York: Free Press.

Stevens, Rosemary. 1971. *American Medicine and the Public Interest.* New Haven, CT: Yale University Press.

Stone, Deborah A. (1988) 2012. *Policy Paradox: The Art of Political Decisionmaking.* 3rd ed. New York: W. W. Norton.

Teske, Steve. 2006a. "Congress: Health Care Reform Issues Top Priority in New Congress, House Democrats Say." *BNA Health Care Policy Report* (November 13).

———. 2006b. "Congress: Congressional Aides Predict Busy Year for Health Care Initiatives in 2007." *BNA Health Care Policy Report* (December 18).

———. 2007a. "SCHIP: Various Groups Seek SCHIP Changes as Finance Committee Prepares for Markup." *BNA Health Care Policy Report* (May 28).

———.2007b. "SCHIP: Senate Finance Markup of SCHIP Bill Possible Week of June 11, Baucus Says." *BNA Health Care Policy Report* (June 11).

———. 2007c. "SCHIP: Finance Panel's Tentative Agreement Would Fund Reauthorization with Tobacco Tax Hike." *BNA Health Care Policy Report* (July 16).

———. 2007d. "SCHIP: Senate Vote on Bill Likely Week of July 23, Despite Bush Veto Threat, Sponsors Say." *BNA Health Care Policy Report* (July 23).

———. 2007e. "New Policies Aimed at Stopping 'Crowd-Out' Anger States, Child Advocacy Groups." *BNA Health Care Policy Report* (August 27).

———. 2007f. "SCHIP: Senate, House Democratic Leaders Seek to Forge Compromise SCHIP Legislation." *BNA Health Care Policy Report* (September 10).

———. 2007g. "SCHIP: House May Have to Drop Some Medicare Provisions to Reach Deal, Rep. Pallone Says." *BNA Health Care Policy Report* (September 17).

———. 2007h. "SCHIP: Bush Urges 'Clean' Bill, Blames Democrats If Veto Leads to Children Losing Coverage." *BNA Health Care Policy Report* (September 24).

———. 2007i. "SCHIP: Congress Passes $35 Billion SCHIP Bill but President Promises Veto, Citing Cost." *BNA Health Care Policy Report* (October 1).

———. 2007j. "SCHIP: AMA, AARP Urge House Lawmakers to Vote to Override President's SCHIP Veto." *BNA Health Care Policy Report* (October 15).

———. 2007k. "SCHIP: Senate Approves Reauthorization Bill: Negotiations with House GOP to Continue." *BNA Health Care Policy Report* (November 5).

———. 2007l. "Medicare: Congress Approves Medicare/SCHIP Bill to Boost Doctor Pay, Extend SCHIP to 2009." *BNA Health Care Policy Report* (December 24).

———. 2008. "Lawmakers Cite GAO, CRS Findings in Faulting CMS's 2007 Enrollment Directive." *BNA Health Care Policy Report* (April 28).

Teske, Steve, and Terence Hyland. 2007. "SCHIP: Senate, House Pass SCHIP Legislation Despite Strong Objection from White House." *BNA Health Care Policy Report* (August 6).

Teske, Steve, and Jonathan Nicholson. 2007a. "SCHIP: After Failure of SCHIP Override Vote, Pelosi Vows to Send Bush Another Similar Bill." *BNA Health Care Policy Report* (October 22).

———. 2007b. "SCHIP: House Fails to Find Veto-Proof Majority on Revised Version of SCHIP Legislation." *BNA Health Care Policy Report* (October 29).

Teske, Steve, and Kendra Casey Plank. 2007. "SCHIP/Medicare: One House Panel Approves Its Part of SCHIP/Medicare Bill, as Work Continues." *BNA Health Care Policy Report* (July 30).

Thompson, Frank J. 1998. "The Faces of Devolution." In *Medicaid and Devolution, A View from the States,* edited by Frank J. Thompson and John J. Dilulio. Washington, DC: Brookings Institution Press.

———. 2012. *Medicaid Politics: Federalism, Policy Durability, and Health Reform.* Washington, DC: Georgetown University Press.

Tompkins, Calvin. 1989. "Profiles: A Sense of Urgency." *The New Yorker*, March 27.

USA Today. 1997. "Senate Just Blows Smoke with Anti-Tobacco Tax Talk." May 23.

Washington Post. 1997. "Muscle in the Senate." August 15.

Weiland, Morgan. 2008. "SCHIP: House Fails to Override SCHIP Veto; Democrats Vow to Seek Reauthorization." *BNA Health Care Policy Report* (January 28).

Weisman, Jonathan. 2013. "Violence Act Returns in Test of Republicans' Appeal to Women." *New York Times,* February 4.

Williams, Loretta Morris, and Anne Harrison-Clark. 1989. "Advocacy for Healthy Births." *Women and Health* 15 (3): 101–105.

Wilson, A. L. 1989. "Development of the U.S. Federal Role in Children's Health Care: A Critical Appraisal." In *Children and Health Care: Moral and Social Issues,* edited by L. M. Kopelman and J. C. Moskop. Norwell, MA: Kluwer Academic Publishers.

Woolf, Steven H., and Laudan Aron, eds. 2013. *U.S. Health in International Perspective: Shorter Lives, Poorer Health.* Washington, DC: National Academies Press.

Zahariadis, Nikolaos. 1996. "Selling British Rail: An Idea Whose Time Has Come?" *Comparative Political Studies* 29: 400–422.

Zuckerman, Stephen, and Cynthia Perry. 2007. "Concerns About Parents Dropping Employer Coverage to Enroll in SCHIP Overlook Issues of Affordability." Urban Institute (September). http://www.urban.org/UploadedPDF/411555_schip_overlook.pdf.

Index

Abortion: CHAP failure, 28; delinking from child health issues, 32; partisan clash over social values, 41
Access to health care: SCHIP/CHIP improving access, 143–144 Activist community in Progressive Era, 18
Acute care children's hospitals, 34–35
Adolescent pregnancy, 151
Adult coverage: childless adults, 81, 90–91, 99–100; decline with increasing coverage of children, 141–142; NHIS survey, 153(n2); partisan discord over SCHIPRA reauthorization, 79–80; SCHIP reauthorization, 84–85; Senate Finance Committee reauthorization agreement, 90
Adult health, childhood and, 3
Advisory Council on Social Security, 54
Advocacy groups and coalitions, 6; competing advocacy coalition, 40–42; framing SCHIP expansion, 12, 124; Hatch-Kennedy bill and cigarette tax, 72; response to August 17 directive, 98; Steiner's survey of, 26; structure and dynamics, 10–12. *See also* Children's health advocacy
Affordability of premiums, 84
Affordable Care Act (ACA; 2010), 5–6, 113, 140, 145; impact on CHIP and child health care, 145–147
African Americans: Edelman, Marian Wright, 8, 15, 26–27; infant mortality rate, 148–149

Agenda-setting process, 15–16, 50
Aid to Families with Dependent Children (AFDC), 31
American Academy of Pediatrics (AAP): block grant proposal, 60; children's health policy network, 39; EPSDT enactment, 46(n2); expanding private coverage of children, 54; Medicaid eligibility expansion, 33–34; pregnant women's coverage under SCHIP, 111; SCHIP reauthorization support, 107–109
American Association of Retired Persons (AARP), 107
American Medical Association (AMA): core child advocacy groups, 34; opposing the Sheppard-Towner Act, 18; reauthorization support, 107; SCHIP expansion, 134(n16)
America's Promise Alliance, 106
Anne E. Casey Foundation, 106
Antipoverty movement: CDF origins, 26
Arizona Republican, 131–132
Association of Maternal and Child Health Programs (AMCHP), 33
Atlantic Philanthropies, 106
August 17 directive, 93–94, 120–121

Balanced Budget Act (1997), 3, 49, 53–54, 65–66, 140
Baucus, Max: ACA-CHIP link, 145; adult coverage, 85; framing SCHIP

171

expansion, 119; funding and SCHIP reauthorization, 89; PhRMA support for SCHIP expansion, 110; SCHIP reauthorization provisions, 100–101
"Benchmark" benefit plans, 66
Bennett, Robert, 69
Bentsen, Lloyd, 8, 28, 32
Bilheimer, Linda, 71
Bingaman, Jeff, 106, 113–114
Bipartisanship: CHC support, 129; First Focus, 106–107; Hatch-Kennedy bill strategy, 68–70; March of Dimes, 111–112; Senate Finance Committee debates over reauthorization, 89–91. *See also* Block grant proposal; Hatch-Kennedy bill; Partisanship
Birth defects, 36
Bliley, Thomas Jr., 74(n6)
Block grant proposal, 38–39, 52, 59–66, 109, 138
Blue Cross and blue Shield PPO plan, 66
Bond, Christopher "Kit," 129
Bonilla, Henry, 129
Boren amendment, 61
Budget Act (1974), 52
Budget process, 52–53
Burgess, Michael C., 84
Bush (George H.W.) administration: coverage of adults, 54; funding and eligibility levels, 82–84
Bush (George W.) administration: CHIPRA veto, 96–97; CMS directive, 94, 98–99; community health centers, 21, 129; coverage of pregnant women, 85; framing strategies, 13; opposition to health reform, 126; opposition to SCHIP expansion, 110; partisan discord over SCHIP reauthorization, 79; policy foreshadowing, 10; public-private boundary, 73; reauthorization process, 88; SCHIP veto, 96–97, 139; vetoing SCHIP reauthorization, 2

Campaign for Children's Health, 109–110
Campbell, Ben Nighthorse, 69
Carter administration: CHAP failure, 28; community health centers, 21
Castle, Michael N., 44
Catholic Charities USA, 112
Catholic Church: opposition to the Sheppard-Towner Act, 18
Center for Budget and Policy Priorities, 112

Center for Children and Families, Georgetown University, 87, 106–107, 112
Centers for Medicare and Medicaid Services (CMS), 93–94, 98–99
Chafee, John: advocacy groups supporting Senate bill, 77(n58); BBA conference committee negotiations, 65; block grant proposal, 60–62; Chafee-Rockefeller proposal, 51; Clinton's Health Security plan, 55; death of, 73; political stance, 77(n61); son's appointment, 77(n62)
Chafee, Lincoln, 77(n62)
Chafee-Rockefeller proposal, 61–62
Chicago Tribune, 131
Child Development Group of Mississippi, 26–27
Child Health Assessment Program (CHAP), 28
Child Health Insurance and Lower Deficit (CHILD) Act: provisions, 52; Senate negotiations, 62, 68–69; values framing SCHIP, 71; working families frame, 117
Child health services: history of federally funded programs, 17–22
Child mortality, and WIC programs combating, 21
Child welfare movement, 19
Childless adults, 81, 90–91, 99–100
Children: lack of political resources, 12; moral obligation to, 4; representing innocence, 14
Children First group, 56, 73
Children's Bureau, 19, 23(n11), 103(n21)
The Children's Cause (Steiner), 26
Children's Defense Fund (CDF): appeals to social justice and morality, 15; block grant proposal, 52, 59–66; child welfare under Reagan, 29; Children's Health Group, 107; children's health policy network, 39; Hatch-Kennedy bill, 67, 71–72; maternal and child health coalition, 33; Medicaid eligibility expansion, 32; origins and purpose, 26–27; partisanship of, 106; policy entrepreneurship, 50; Steiner's survey of advocacy groups, 26
Children's Dental Health Improvement Act (2007), 114–115
Children's Dental Health Project (CDHP), 1, 113–114
Children's health advocacy: baseline description, 25–26; CDF and CHAP,

26–28; core advocacy groups, 33–36; framing SCHIP expansion, 124; SCHIP reauthorization, 88–89, 107–111
Children's Health and Medicare Protection Act (CHAMP; 2007), 91–92
Children's Health Group, 107–109
Children's Health Insurance Program Reauthorization Act (CHIPRA), 95, 101, 112–113. *See also* Reauthorization of SCHIP
Children's Investment Fund, 106
Chiles, Lawton, 8, 28
Chronic conditions, 35, 149
Cigarette tax. *See* Tobacco tax
Civic associations, 47(n22)
Civil rights movement: CDF origins, 26; child health policy network emerging from, 39–40
Clinton, Hillary Rodham, 83
Clinton administration: BBA and Reconciliation Acts, 49, 65–66; block grant proposal, 38, 59–66; children's health advocacy, 74(n3); coverage of pregnant women, 85; Hatch-Kennedy bill, 67; health plan failure, 8–9, 55–56, 75(n12), 127; maternal and child health coalition, 40; outreach and enrollment, 81; reducing uninsured children numbers, 51; universal health coverage, 54–55
Coburn, Tom, 3
Collins, Martha Layne, 44
Collins, Susan, 69
Committee for Economic Development (CED), 31, 44, 47(n28)
Community health centers (CHCs), 21, 129
Competing advocacy coalition, 40–42
Congress: attacks on Child Development Group of Misissppi, 26–27; block grant proposal, 59–66; Bush vetoing SCHIP reauthorization, 2; consensus over SCHIP, 49–50; discord over Clinton plan, 55–56; framing strategies, 13; House Select Committee on Children, Youth, and Families, 29–30; interview process, 16–17; March of Dimes nonpartisan reputation, 36; Medicaid eligibility expansion, 31–32; Medicaid expansion as solution to infant mortality, 45; National Commission to Prevent Infant Mortality, 30–31; partisan clash over social values, 41–42; partisan makeup of 110th Congress, 102(n4); policy entrepreneurs within, 28; policy streams model, 7; Progressive Era child health activism, 18; response to August 17 directive, 98–99; SCHIP Medicaid provisions, 94–95; Southern Regional Task Force on Infant Mortality, 30
Congressional hearings: analyzing, 130; dental care coverage, 115; frames used in "Covering the Uninsured Through the Eyes of a Child," 121(table); framing SCHIP expansion, 116, 123–124. *See also specific committees*
Conrad, Kent, 89–90
Contract with America, 59
Core child health advocacy groups, 33–36
Cost-effectiveness frame, 138; coverage of pregnant women and immigrants, 135(n43), 136(n48); future-oriented frame, 118–119; media framing public-private boundary debate, 130–131; prenatal care as, 44–45
Crapo, Mike, 91
Crowd-out: CMS August 17 directive, 93–94; funding and eligibility debate, 82–84; House and Senate reauthorization bills, 92–93; SCHIP reauthorization provisions, 101; Senate Finance Committee debate, 62
Culture wars frame, 127–130

D'Amato, Alfonse, 62
Daschle, Tom, 51, 113
David and Lucile Packard Foundation, 106
Death rate: US versus other high-income nations, 151
Decision agenda, 50–54
Deficit Reduction Act, 31
Delivery of child health services, 144; advocacy coalitions shaping policy, 12; NACHRI, 34–35; SCHIP reauthorization, 112–113 Dental coverage: CHIPRA provision, 102; conservative opposition, 134(n35); Deamonte Driver's death, 1, 114–115, 122, 134(n33); framing SCHIP expansion, 121–122; reauthorization debate over, 88, 92; SCHIP reauthorization, 113–115; US health status, 149–150
Department of Health, Education, and Welfare (DHEW), 20, 23(n11)

174 Index

Department of Health and Human Services (DHHS): opposition to SCHIP expansion, 126–127; quality of care measurement, 101, 112–113; response to August 17 directive, 98; Senate Finance Committee reauthorization agreement, 90
Dependent groups, 14
Development, childhood: importance of good health, 3; pediatrics and the child welfare movement, 19
Diarrhea, 17–18
Dingell, John, 83, 89, 134(n18)
Distributive programs, 3–4
Dodd, Christopher, 46(n4), 56, 75(n13)
Dominant advocacy coalition, 39
DREAM Act, 14
Driver, Deamonte, 1, 114–115, 122, 134(n33)

Early Periodic Screening, Diagnosis, and Treatment (EPSDT): BBA conference committee negotiations, 65–66; Clinton plan failure, 55; creation of, 20; dental care through CHIP, 113; effectiveness of advocacy groups, 26; enactment factors, 46(n2); exclusion from Johnson-Matsui bill, 64; federal block grant proposal, 61; implementation, 37–38; Kennedy-Hatch bill, 63; NGA opposition to, 59
Economic framing , 15, 43, 135(n40)
Edelman, Marian Wright, 8, 15, 26
Edelstein, Burton L., 113, 115, 134(n30)
Education/investment frame, 118, 120, 122–123, 130–131. *See also* Investment in the future frame
Elderly population, 75(n14); Medicaid eligibility expansion, 32; Medicaid shift from children to, 21
Elections: limiting expansion through entitlement, 139; shifting political streams, 145; 2008 election and SCHIP reauthorization, 99
Emergency Maternity and Infant Care Program, 20
Emphasis framing, 13
Employer-based coverage: House and Senate reauthorization bills, 92
Enrollment: AAP support for, 108–109; CHAMP Act, 91–92; First Focus advocacy, 107; increasing children's enrollment, 141–142; reauthorization debate, 87–88; simplification and outreach, 81
Entitlement: Kennedy-Hatch bill as, 68–69
Expansion of SCHIP: framing, 115–125; framing the opposition to, 125–133. *See also* Reauthorization of SCHIP

Families USA: children's health policy network, 39; core child advocacy groups, 36; immigrants' coverage under SCHIP, 112; Medicaid and SCHIP expansion, 33, 109–110, 134(n16)
Family and marriage: culture war framing opposition to SCHIP expansion, 127–128; National Commission on Children's view of child health, 41–42
Family and medical leave, 34
Family Values Child Health Insurance Act, 58
Federal poverty level (FPL): ACA expansion, 145; Bush's proposed funding and eligibility levels, 82; Medicaid eligibility expansion, 32; state use of federal money, 81
Federally funded programs: community health centers, 21; history of, 17–19; retrenchment in the 1970ƨ, 21–22; Steiner's survey of, 26. *See also* Medicaid
First Focus, 106–107, 112
Focusing events, 7, 114–115, 122
Ford Foundation, 31, 44–45
Framing effects, 13, 115–125
Framing strategies, 5; children and children's issues, 12–15; children's advocacy groups, 12; cost effectiveness and solvability, 43–45; defining, 22(n5); economic framing, 15; investment in children's health, 42–46; media frame of public-private boundary debate, 130–133, 136(nn60,61); opposition to SCHIP expansion, 125–133. *See also* Cost-effectiveness frame; Economic framing; Future-oriented frame; Hard-working frame; Human capital frame; Innocence frame; Morality frame; Worthiness frame
Funding: CHIPRA provisions, 101; scope of Bush proposal, 82–84; shortfall issues, 86–87. *See also* Tobacco tax
Future-oriented frame, 116–120

Galen Institute, 82

General Accounting Office (GAO), 103(n20)
George Gund Foundation, 106
Gingrich, Newt, 36, 59, 129
Gormley, William T., Jr., 124, 135(n40), 152, 153(n1)
Government Accountability Office (GAO), 98, 103(n20)
Governors: framing SCHIP expansion, 122–123. *See also* National Governors Association; State government
Governors' Conference, 37
Gramm, Phil, 51, 62
Grant-in-aid programs, 18
Grassley, Charles: adult coverage, 84–85; Bush veto of CHIPRA, 95–96, 103(n6); PhRMA support for SCHIP reauthorization, 110; SCHIP reauthorization debate, 89; SCHIP reauthorization provisions, 100–101; tobacco tax, 83
Great Depression, 19–20
Gregoire, Christine, 123
Gun regulation, 34–35

Hard-working families frame, 71, 116–117, 121–122
Harkin, Tom, 55–56, 75(n14)
Hatch, Orrin: block grant proposal, 60; Bush veto of CHIPRA, 96; Chafee amendment, 62; cigarette tax, 53; conservatives' pleas for free market reforms, 83; outreach and enrollment, 87; policy entrepreneurship, 9, 50; SCHIP reauthorization, 89–90; SCHIP reauthorization provisions, 101; shortfall issues, 87; "working families" frame, 117
Hatch-Kennedy bill, 51–52; bipartisan involvement, 68–70; Chafee-Rockefeller bill and, 61; controversy over, 60–61; framing strategies, 70–73; Kerry-Kennedy bill and, 76(42); marketing the proposal, 70–73; Senate Finance Committee debate, 62; terms of, 67
Health disadvantage, 151
Health insurance plans, 54
Health Insurance Portability and Accountability Act (1996), 68
Health maintenance organization (HMO), 66
Health Security plan, 55–56

Health status: effectiveness of SCHIP/CHIP, 144; US and other wealthy nations, 140–141, 148–153
Health Subcommittee, House Ways and Means Committee, 63–64
Health Subcommittee, Senate Finance Committee, 98
Healthcare reform, 126–127
Heritage Foundation, 82–84, 127
Hispanics: infant mortality rate, 148–149; SCHIP reauthorization provisions, 100
Hooley, Darlene, 122
Hospitals. *See* National Association of Children's Hospitals and Related Institutions
House: CHIPRA veto, 96–97; passage of SCHIP reauthorization bill, 99–100
House Committee on Energy and Commerce, 74(n4); CMS directives, 98; dental coverage, 115; framing SCHIP expansion, 121; jurisdictional disputes, 52; Medicaid block grant bill, 64–65; Medicaid jurisdiction, 74(nn5,6); OTA strategies on children's health, 43; school-based health centers, 41
House Select Committee on Children, Youth, and Families, 29–30, 42, 154(n7)
House Ways and Means Committee: coverage for pregnant women, 54; jurisdictional disputes, 52; Medicaid block grant bill, 63–64; Medicaid jurisdiction, 74(nn5,6); reauthorization debate, 91
Houston Chronicle, 132
Human capital frame, 118, 135(n43)
Hyde, Henry, 32

Ideology: Bush vetoing SCHIP reauthorization, 2–3, 139; CMS August 17 directive, 94; consensus over SCHIP, 49–50; framing opposition to SCHIP expansion, 126–127; framing strategies, 15; media framing public-private boundary debate, 130–133; partisan and ideological conflict over reauthorization, 4–5
Immigrants: CHIPRA veto over, 97; cost-effective frame, 135(n43); coverage under SCHIP, 112; partisan debate over, 86; reauthorization provision, 103(n8); SCHIP reauthorization provisions, 100–101;

Senate Finance Committee reauthorization agreement, 90
Immunization, 2, 36, 42
Implementation of SCHIP, 5, 152
Income eligibility: CHIPRA veto, 96–97; CMS August 17 directive, 93–94; Senate and House bills, 92–93; Senate Finance Committee debate, 89–91
Incrementalism: Children First proposal, 56; Hatch-Kennedy bill strategy, 68; linking children's health insurance to universal health coverage, 139; pregnant women and children, 74–75(n10); SCHIP as step in, 125–126
Industrialization: child health advocacy, 17–18
Infant milk stations, 17–18
Infant mortality: framing Medicaid eligibility expansion, 42–43; health services for pregnant women and children, 154(n7); metric of usefulness, 154(n7); National Commission to Prevent Infant Mortality, 30–31; prenatal care link, 43–45; Progressive Era, 17–18; Southern Regional Task Force on Infant Mortality, 30; US health status, 2, 148–149; US versus other high-income nations, 151, 154(n9)
Ingram, Helen, 6, 13, 14
Innocence frame, 14, 130–131
Institute of Medicine, 44, 119, 141, 144, 150–151, 153
Institutional agenda, 50
Interest groups: competing advocacy coalition, 40–42; culture war framing opposition to SCHIP expansion, 127–128; framing strategies, 13; interview process, 16–17; maternal and child health coalition, 33–34; policy community representation, 11–12
Interview process, 15–17
Investment in the future frame, 122–123, 136(n48)

Jeffords, James, 62, 69, 73
Johnson, Kay A., 28
Johnson, Lyndon, 80
Johnson, Nancy L., 51, 64, 70–71
Johnson-Matsui bill, 64

Kaiser Foundation, 106, 114
Kassebaum, Nancy, 68

Kennedy, Edward: block grant proposal, 39, 52, 59–66, 109, 138; CHC support, 129; cigarette tax, 53; Clinton's Health Security plan, 55; Family Values Child Health Insurance Act, 58; framing SCHIP expansion, 119–120; Hatch-Kennedy bill, 51–52; immigration reform, 86; policy entrepreneurship, 9, 50; tobacco tax, 74(n7); "working families" frame, 117. *See also* Hatch-Kennedy bill
Kerry, John, 57–58, 68
Kerry-Kennedy bill, 69, 71, 76(n42)
Kingdon, John, 6–9

League of Women Voters, 18
Leave No Child Behind, 27
Leavitt, Michael O., 61, 90, 127
Leland, Mickey, 32
Lesley, Bruce, 124
Lott, Trent, 69, 90
Low birth weight, 149
Low-income families: CDF research, 27; Clinton plan, 55–56; Families USA, 36; House Select Committee on Children, Youth, and Families, 29–30; impact of ACA on CHIP, 145–146; Medicaid eligibility expansion, 31–32; Medicaid provision of preventive care, 20; opposition to the Sheppard-Towner Act, 19; Southern Regional Task Force on Infant Mortality, 30; uninsured children, 50–54; US health status, 149

"Maintenance of effort" provision of ACA, 147–148
Majority Report of chapter on health (National Commission on Children), 54
Malnourishment, 29
Mandatory coverage, 55–56, 102
Mann, Cindy, 83
March of Dimes: children's health policy network, 39; coverage of pregnant women, 85–86, 111; immigrants' coverage under SCHIP, 112; maternal and child health coalition, 34; Medicaid eligibility expansion, 33; SCHIP reauthorization and expansion, 108
Marketing policy. *See* Framing strategies
Massachusetts: state child health insurance bill, 58
Maternal and child health coalition, 33; AAP, 33–34, 38, 40; CDF, 26, 28, 32, 33; children's health policy network,

Index   **177**

38–42; Families USA, 36; March of Dimes, 34; NACHRI, 34–35; National Governors Association, 37. *See also under individual groups*
Maternity and Infancy Act. *See* Sheppard-Towner Act
Matsui, Robert, 51, 54, 64
McDonough, John, 58
Media: Deamonte Driver death, 114–115; driving public policy, 1; Edelman's CDF advocacy, 27; focusing events, 7; Hatch-Kennedy bill and cigarette tax, 72–73; PhRMA campaign for SCHIP expansion, 110; public-private boundary debate, 130–133; SCHIP expansion, 134(n16), 136(nn60,61)
Medicaid: block grant proposal, 59–66; enactment of, 20; increase in uninsured children, 50–51; interview process, 15–16; NACHRI services, 35; NHIS survey, 153(n2); policy entrepreneurship and the expansion of, 8; Reagan administration funding cuts, 28–29; reducing uninsured children numbers, 51; retrenchment in the 1970s, 21–22. *See also* Block grant proposal
Medicaid and CHIP Payment and Access Commission (MACPAC), 113
Medicaid eligibility expansion: Chafee amendment, 62–63; Commerce Committee bill, 64–65; core child advocacy groups, 33–36; delinking abortion from, 42; emergence of the child health advocacy community, 25; federal block grant proposal, 61; framing strategies, 70; increasing uninsured children numbers, 57; maternal and child health coalition, 37; Reagan-era efforts, 31–32; reducing uninsured children numbers, 52; shifting emphasis from infants to children, 42–43; Southern Regional Task Force on Infant Mortality, 30
Medicaid medical industrial complex, 128
Medicare: political connections to child health policy, 5–6
Mental illness, 3
Migration: Progressive Era child health advocacy, 17
Military service: World War II prenatal care programs, 20
Miller, Bob, 61
Miller, George E., 8, 28–29, 32

Minority Chapter of the National Commission on Children, 40–41
Mitchell, George J., 55, 75(n13)
Montana: framing SCHIP expansion, 124–125; "working families" frame, 117–118
Morality frame: CDF activities, 27; Edelman's use of, 135(n40); framing opposition to SCHIP expansion, 127–128; framing SCHIP expansion, 116, 120, 123–125; Hatch-Kennedy bill and cigarette tax, 72; media framing public-private boundary debate, 130–131; morality-compassion frame, 122
Murtha, John, 114

National Association of Children's Hospitals and Related Institutions (NACHRI): block grant proposal, 60; children's health policy network, 39; EPSDT support, 38; maternal and child health coalition, 34–35; Medicaid eligibility expansion, 33; origins and growth of, 46(n15); SCHIP reauthorization and expansion, 108
National Association of Community Health Centers (NACHC), 32, 46(n9)
National Commission on Children, 40–41, 54
National Commission to Prevent Infant Mortality, 42–45, 138
National Council of La Raza (NCLR), 112
National Foundation for Infantile Paralysis, 34
National Governors Association (NGA): block grant proposal, 61, 64–65; children's health policy network, 39; dental coverage, 134(n35); EPSDT opposition, 59; framing cost-effectiveness and solvability of infant mortality, 44; maternal and child health coalition, 37; Medicaid eligibility expansion, 33; oral health coverage, 114; SCHIP reauthorization, 99; shortfall issues, 87; Southern Regional Task Force on Infant Mortality, 30
National health insurance, 127. *See also* Public-private boundary
National Health Interview Survey (NHIS), 153(n2)
National Immigration Law Center (NILC), 112
National Research Council, 150–151

National Welfare Rights Organization, 26
New Jersey: response to August 17 directive, 98
New York City Bureau of Child Hygiene, 18
New York Times, 130, 134(n16)
Nickles, Don, 62
Nixon administration, 26–27
No Child Left Behind, 27
Nontraditional healthcare delivery, 113
Nutrition: WIC program, 21

Obama administration: community health centers, 21; SCHIP reauthorization, 2, 99
Obamacare. *See* Affordable Care Act
Obesity: framing investment in children's health, 3, 42, 124; PhRMA issues, 110–111; US health disadvantage, 151; US statistics, 149
Office of Technology Assessment (OTA), 31, 43
Oliver, Thomas, 22(n3)
Olson, Laura Katz, 128
Omnibus Budget Reconciliation Act (1989), 38
Oral health. *See* Dental coverage
Oral Health in America report, 114
Outreach provision, 81, 87–88
Owcharenko, Nina, 82

Pallone, Frank, Jr., 51
Partisanship: ACA implementation, 147; adult coverage, 84–85; BBA conference committee negotiations, 65; Bush's reauthorization veto, 2–3; competing advocacy coalition, 40; discord over SCHIP enactment, 49–50; discord over SCHIP reauthorization, 79; EPSDT, 37–38; failure of block grant proposal, 64–65; funding and eligibility debate, 82–83; ideological opposition to SCHIP expansion, 127–130; immigrants' coverage, 86; implementation of ACA and CHIP, 152; interview process, 16–17; March of Dimes nonpartisan reputation, 36; opposition to the Hatch-Kennedy bill, 69–70; partisan and ideological conflict over reauthorization, 4–5, 91; reducing uninsured children numbers, 51. *See also* Bipartisanship
Patient Protection and Affordable Care Act. *See* Affordable Care Act

Patrick, Deval L., 123
Pear, Robert, 56, 134(n16)
Pediatrics: child welfare movement, 19; Medicaid eligibility expansion, 33–34; pediatricians' role in social policy, 23(n10)
Pence, Mike, 126
Perdue, Sonny, 84, 123
Personal Responsibility and Work Opportunity Reconciliation Act (PRWORA; 1996), 74(n3), 86
Peterson, Mark, 9
PhRMA (Pharmaceutical Research and Manufacturers of America), 110–111, 128, 134(nn16,18)
Physicians: opposition to the Sheppard-Towner Act, 18–19. *See also* American Academy of Pediatrics; American Medical Association
Pierson, Paul, 9–10
Policy actors/policy community: actors in the child health policy network, 38–42; advocacy coalitions, 10–12; baseline description of child health policy, 26; Edelman and the CDF, 26–28; emergence of the child health advocacy community, 2, 25; framing strategies, 13; future-oriented frame for SCHIP expansion, 121; interview process, 15–17; policy streams model, 7; political stream interaction, 138–139; punctuated equilibrium model, 139–140. *See also* Congress; Policy entrepreneurs; Private organizations; Public institutions
Policy agenda, 54–58
Policy entrepreneurs: CDF, 28; emergence of the child health advocacy community, 25; Medicaid expansion as solution to infant mortality, 45–46; policy streams model, 7–8; state and federal level insurance bills, 58. *See also* Kennedy, Edward
Policy foreshadowing, 10
Policy legacies, 10, 45, 116, 137–138. *See also* Social learning
Policy monopoly, 140
Policy network. *See* Policy actors/policy community
Policy process: advocacy coalitions, 6, 10–12; block grant proposal, 59–66; defining the problem at state and federal levels, 56–58; discord over SCHIP enactment, 49–50; policy

legacies, 6, 9–11; policy streams model, 6–9; social construction of target populations, 6. *See also* Framing strategies
Policy research, 11
Policy streams model, 6–9
Polio, 34
Political resources: children's lack of, 12; NACHRI, 35–36
Political stream, 7–9, 55, 73, 99, 102, 139, 145
Powell, Colin, 106
Preexisting conditions, 146
Preferred provider organization (PPO) plan, 66
Pregnant women: adolescent pregnancy statistics, 151; adult coverage under SCHIP, 85; CHAP failure, 28; Children First proposal, 56; cost-effective frame, 135(n43); employee health insurance, 54; incremental strategies towards universal coverage, 139; Kerry-Kennedy bill and Hatch-Kennedy bill, 76(42); maternal and child health coalition, 33; Medicaid eligibility expansion, 31–32; Medicaid expansion, 2–3, 8; Medicaid shift from children to the elderly, 21; Mitchell bill, 75(n13); partisan debate over SCHIP reauthorization, 85–86; passage of SCHIP reauthorization bill, 99–100; SCHIP reauthorization provisions, 100–101, 111; Senate and House bills, 92; Senate Finance Committee reauthorization agreement, 90; World War II prenatal care programs, 20. *See also* Medicaid eligibility expansion; Prenatal care
Premature births, 36
Prenatal care: House Select Committee on Children, Youth, and Families, 29–30; preventing low birth weight and infant mortality, 43–44; Southern Regional Task Force on Infant Mortality, 30. *See also* Pregnant women
Preventive health care: ACA requirement, 146; CHIPRA dental provision, 102; House Select Committee on Children, Youth, and Families, 29–30; Medicaid enactment, 20; Title V, 20; US health status, 149–150
Private health sector: ACA provisions for children, 146; affordability of premiums, 84; children's loss of coverage, 57; expanding children's coverage through, 54; opposition to Clinton plan, 55–56; outreach and enrollment, 81; partisan and ideological conflict over reauthorization, 4; SCHIP enrollment provision, 128
Private organizations: CDF funding, 27; children's health policy network, 39; children's health policy recommendations, 31; framing opposition to SCHIP expansion, 128; maternal and child health coalition, 33
Problem stream, 7
Progressive Era, child health advocacy in the, 17–19
Public health sector: children with public plan coverage, 141(fig.); partisan and ideological conflict over reauthorization, 4
Public institutions: child health policy network, 39; emergence in the 1980s, 29–31; House Select Committee on Children, Youth, and Families, 29–30; National Commission to Prevent Infant Mortality, 30–31; Southern Regional Task Force on Infant Mortality, 30
Public opinion, framing and, 13–14. *See also* Framing strategies
Public-private boundary: Bush opposition to reauthorization, 79; Bush veto of CHIPRA, 95; CMS August 17 directive, 94; community health center programs, 129–130; media framing, 130–133, 136(n59)
Punctuated equilibrium model, 139–140

Quality of service: DHHS measurement provision, 101, 112–113, 144; House and Senate reauthorization bills, 92; US health status, 150

Reagan administration: competing advocacy coalition, 40–41; House Select Committee on Children, Youth, and Families, 29–30; Medicaid cuts, 28–29; National Commission to Prevent Infant Mortality, 30–31; social movements and child health policy, 39–40
Reauthorization of SCHIP: adult coverage, 84–85; advocacy groups, 105–107; August 17 directive, 93–94; Bush vetoing, 2–3, 95–97, 139; CHAMP Act, 91–92; CHIPRA, 95, 101, 112–113;

dental care coverage, 113–115; final provisions, 99–103; funding and eligibility, 82–84, 103(n12); House Ways and Means Committee debate, 91; ideological polarization, 139; as incremental expansion step, 125–126; issues of controversy, 80–88; legal immigrants, 86; Medicaid provisions, 94–95; nomenclature, 17; outreach and enrollment, 87–88; partisan and ideological conflict over, 4–5, 79–80; pregnant women's coverage, 85–86; Senate and House bills, 91–93; Senate Finance Committee debate, 89–91; shifting social policy, 4–5; shortfall issues, 86–87; supportive coalitions, 107–111; as window of opportunity, 111

Reconciliation process, 52–53

Reform movements, 22(n4)

Reimbursement: Affordable Care Act, 113; Boren amendment, 61, 66; coverage of pregnant women, 85; House and Senate reauthorization bills, 91–92; reauthorization debate, 90–91; reauthorization extension, 97–98

Religion: Catholic Charities USA, 112; Catholic Church's opposition to the Sheppard-Towner Act, 18; Edelman's advocacy, 27; immigrants' coverage under SCHIP, 112; US Conference of Catholic Bishops, 46(n10)

Representational groups, 39

Reproductive health: culture war framing opposition to SCHIP expansion, 127–128; partisan clash over social values, 41

Research methodology, 15–17, 116–117, 153(n3)

Revenue Reconciliation Act (1997), 3, 49, 140

Riley, Richard W., 8, 30, 37

Robert Wood Johnson Foundation, 81, 106, 113

Roberts, Pat, 90, 101

Rockefeller, John A. "Jay": ACA-CHIP link, 145; advocacy groups supporting Senate bill, 77(n58); block grant proposal, 60; Chafee-Rockefeller proposal, 51; Children First group, 56; response to August 17 directive, 98; SCHIP reauthorization, 89, 101; shortfall issues, 87

Rosenbaum, Sara, 8, 28

Roth, William, 63, 65

Roukema, Marge, 51

Sabatier, Paul A., 11

Schneider, Anne, 6, 13, 14

School-based health care, 41, 113

Seat belt regulation, 34–35

Senate: CHIPRA veto, 96–97; passage of SCHIP reauthorization bill, 99–100

Senate Children's Caucus, 46(n4)

Senate Finance Committee: ACA-CHIP link, 145; adult coverage under SCHIP, 84–85; CMS directives, 98; competing health plan proposals, 62–63; coverage of pregnant women, 85–86; framing SCHIP expansion, 117, 119; funding and SCHIP reauthorization, 89; Hatch advocacy, 69; SCHIP enactment, 52; SCHIP reauthorization, 89–91, 101; shortfall issues, 87; tobacco tax, 53, 70

Senate Labor and Human Resources Committee, 43

September 11, 2001, 14

Sheppard-Towner Act (1921), 18–20, 34

Simpson, Michael, 114

Situational learning, 10, 67, 137–138

Skocpol, Theda, 39, 47(n22), 75(n12)

Smith, Bob, 69

Smith, Gordon, 91

Snowball sampling technique, 16

Snowe, Olympia: CHILD legislation, 69; CHIPRA dental provision, 102; response to August 17 directive, 98; SCHIP reauthorization debate, 91; SCHIP reauthorization provisions, 100

Social learning, 10, 45, 137–138

Social movements, child health policy network emerging from, 39–40

Social policy: partisan and ideological conflict over reauthorization, 4–5; pediatricians' role in, 23(n10)

Social Security Act (1935), 20, 56. *See also* Title V programs

Social values: competing advocacy coalition, 40–42; framing strategies, 15; framing the CHILD and Hatch-Kennedy bills, 71; US health disadvantage stemming from, 151–152

Socialized health care, 3; CHIPRA debate, 95; SCHIP expansion as step towards, 126. *See also* Public-private boundary

Softening up process, 8

Solvability of infant mortality and children's illness, 43–45

Southern Governors' Association, 30, 84–85
Southern Legislative Conference, 30
Southern Regional Task Force on Infant Mortality, 30, 37
Specialization, policy, 11
Spector, Arlen, 46(n4), 51
Stark, Pete, 51, 60
State Children's Health Insurance Program (SCHIP): achievements and limitations of, 140–144; creation of, 49–50; defining the problem at state and federal levels, 56–58; enactment of, 50–54; framing strategies, 70–73; implementation, 5, 152; Medicaid expansion shaping, 38. *See also* Policy actors/policy community; Policy process; Reauthorization of SCHIP
State government: adult coverage, 84–85; BBA plan, 65–66; CHILD Act, 52, 62; cost effectiveness and solvability frames, 44–45; enrollment in CHIP/SCHIP, 141–142; EPSDT, 37–38; exclusion of EPSDT from Johnson-Matsui bill, 64; federal block grant proposal, 61; maintaining CHIP with ACA, 147–148; Medicaid eligibility expansion, 31–32; SCHIP policy relationship, 3; shortfall issues, 86–87; Southern Regional Task Force on Infant Mortality, 30; Title V programs, 19–20; use of SCHIP money, 80–81; "working families" frame, 117–118
Steiner, Gilbert Y., 12, 26
Stevens, Ted, 69
Stone, Deborah, 10, 12
Subcommittee on Health and the Environment, 41, 43, 54
Substantive policy learning, 10, 13, 45
Subsystems, policy, 11
Suffrage, 18

Target populations, 6, 138; historical framing strategies, 13–15
Task Force on National Health Reform, 40
Tauzin, Billy, 110
Tax credits: for higher-income families, 82; Kennedy and CDF opposition, 67
Tax reform, 82–83
Tax revenue, 52–53
Thomas, Bill, 64, 70–71, 74(n6)
Thompson, Frank J., 6, 22(n2) Title V programs: EPSDT enactment, 46(n2); Gramm's expansion proposal, 62;

maternal and child health, 103(n21); reducing uninsured children numbers, 52; Sheppard-Towner Act, 19–20; Steiner's survey of advocacy groups, 26
Tobacco advertising, 34–35
Tobacco tax: Children First proposal, 56; CHIPRA funding, 95; hard-working families frame, 138; Hatch-Kennedy bill, 52, 68–70, 72; opposition to SCHIP expansion, 126; SCHIP reauthorization provisions, 101; Senate and House bills, 92; Senate Finance Committee and the Hatch-Kennedy bill, 74(n7); Senate Finance Committee reauthorization agreement, 90; Senate Finance Committee support, 53; Weld's opposition to, 58
Trojan horse, SCHIP expansion as, 4, 13, 133
Truman, Harry, 56

Unfunded mandates, 38
UNICEF, 151
Uninsured children: ACA and Medicaid/CHIP, 146–147; community health centers, 129; decline from 2008-2011, 142; Medicaid block grant proposal, 63; Medicaid coverage in the 1980s addressing, 57; SCHIP enactment, 50–54; SCHIP reduction of numbers, 81; teens, 74(n2)
Universal health coverage, 2, 4, 54, 139. *See also* Incrementalism; Public-private boundary
Urbanization: Progressive Era child health advocacy, 17–18
US Catholic Conference, 32, 46(n10)
U.S. Health in International Perspective: Shorter Lives, Poorer Health, 150–151, 153
USA Today, 72

Value recruitment, framing as, 12–13
Values. *See* Social values
Veto, presidential: Bush opposition to SCHIP, 126; CHIPRA, 96–97; framing SCHIP expansion, 116; House and Senate reauthorization bills, 90, 93; ideological roots of, 2; media framing public-private boundary debate, 131–132; political stalemate following, 80; SCHIP Medicaid provisions, 94–95
Violence Against Women Act, 22(n1)
Voucher programs, 51, 57–58, 60, 82

Vulnerability of children frame, 117–120, 124–125

War on Poverty, 21
Washington Post, 72–73, 130
Waxman, Henry, 8, 28, 32, 41, 73
Weld, William, 58
Welfare reform, 60
Welfare system increasing uninsured children numbers, 57
Well-baby conferences, 19
White House conferences on children, 18
Window of opportunity, 9; policy streams model, 7; SCHIP reauthorization, 111
Women: decline of civic activity in the Progressive Era, 47(n22); Progressive Era child health activism, 18. *See also* Pregnant women
Women, Infants, and Children (WIC) program, 21, 87–88
Women's Joint Congressional Committee, 18
Workforce: children's health services as investment in, 45, 116–118; decline in employee coverage, 141–142; decline of civic activity, 47(n22); employees' right to health care coverage, 54
Working class: uninsured children, 50–54
Working families frame, 32, 57–58, 70–73, 83, 116–123, 121(table), 130, 135(n45)
Worthiness frame, 4, 25, 42, 138
Wright, F. Vernon, 117

About the Book

Assuring that low-income children have health insurance coverage would seem to be a noncontroversial and popular issue. Yet, the policy history of US children's health insurance is full of drama, and the fate of the federal State Children's Health Insurance Program (SCHIP) has been marked by ideological conflict and two presidential vetoes. Why?
   Alice Sardell answers this question through an examination of the policy legacies and decisions that shaped SCHIP, the advocacy strategies that created and sustained it, and the actors who interacted to either support or oppose its expansion. Her analysis illustrates the critical importance of policy entrepreneurs, both inside and outside government, in the US policymaking process.

Alice Sardell is professor in the Department of Urban Studies at Queens College/CUNY. Her previous book is *The U.S. Experiment in Social Medicine: The Community Health Center Program, 1965–1986.*